ROBERT S. MENDELSOHN, M.D., has been practicing pediatrics for almost thirty years. He has been the national director of Project Head Start's Medical Consultation Service, chairman of the Medical Licensing Committee for the State of Illinois, and associate professor of Preventive Medicine and Community Health in the School of Medicine of the University of Illinois. Dr. Mendelsohn has received numerous awards for excellence in medicine and medical instruction.

How to Raise a Healthy Child... In Spite of Your Doctor

Robert S. Mendelsohn, M.D.

BALLANTINE BOOKS • NEW YORK

A Ballantine Book
Published by The Random House Publishing Group

Published in the United States by Ballantine Books, an imprint of The Random House Publishing Group, a division of Random House, Inc., New York, and simultaneously in Canada by Random House of Canada Limited, Toronto.

Ballantine and colophon are registered trademarks of Random House, Inc.

ISBN 0-345-34276-3

www.ballantinebooks.com

This edition published by arrangement with Contemporary Books, Inc.

Manufactured in the United States of America

First Ballantine Books Edition: June 1987

OPM   39   38   37   36   35   34   33   32   31

Contents

Introduction

This book reflects my belief that in pediatrics, as in other specialties, a great deal of bad medicine is practiced in the United States. That does not imply, however, that doctors have less integrity or compassion than the rest of mankind. The shortcomings lie within the philosophy and teaching of medicine, not in the character of those who are taught.

Doctors aren't culprits. Like their patients, they are victims of the system. They are the first to be impaired by medical education's preoccupation with intervention rather than prevention, its infatuation with drugs and technology, and the indefensible rituals, mores, and egotistical attitudes that are burned into the brain of every student who survives the rigid and often irrelevant curriculum and training. They emerge with their heads so stuffed with institutionalized foolishness that there is no room left for common sense.

I don't exempt myself from this criticism of other pediatricians. I confess that I began my medical practice believing most of what I had been taught, and my patients paid the price for many years. Fortunately, perhaps because I began teaching medical students myself, I learned to question many of the medical principles that had been drilled into me and to suspect every new drug, surgical procedure, and medical "innovation" that came along. I soon discovered that most of them couldn't withstand rigorous scientific evaluation and that an incredible percentage of the "wonder drugs" and "revolutionary procedures" soon disappeared when it was discovered that they did more harm than good.

In my two previous books, *Confessions of a Medical Heretic* and *Male Practice*: *How Doctors Manipulate Women*, I sought to caution my readers about the hazards of blind faith in the American medical profession. It was not my purpose then, nor is it now, to discourage my readers from seeking *needed* medical attention. Despite the shortcomings of their education and training, doctors *do* save lives, and they *do* make sick people well. They are at their best when challenged by medical emergencies and at their worst when they feel compelled—as they were taught to do—to treat people who aren't really sick.

I hoped, in those books and this one, to alert you to the deficiencies of medical practice so that you would be prepared to defend yourself against dangerous and inappropriate medical treatment. As a subsidiary objective, I reasoned that if enough patients began to question their doctors about the treatments they prescribed, the doctors might begin to question them, too.

It may be coincidental, and much of the progress must be credited to other critics within and outside my profession, but there is strong evidence that these objectives are being achieved. Many doctors are being prompted by their patients and by the media to question their own medical beliefs. I know this is true, because my colleagues frequently tell me so and because surveys of doctors indicate that a growing number of patients are refusing to take their doctor's opinions at face value.

Patients have become less in awe of their doctors, less docile and compliant. Doctors are no longer—in the minds of many patients—invested with scientific infallibility. Instead, they are being compelled to search for plausible answers to tough questions about the drugs they prescribe, the tests they order, and the surgery they recommend. The impact is great when a doctor repeatedly finds himself looking for defensive answers that aren't there.

Many of the doctors I know welcome these changes, but others find them disconcerting when they are unable to explain or to defend many of the drugs and procedures that they have prescribed routinely in the past. In either case, however, the new awareness of the shortcomings of conventional medical practice is yielding constructive changes. When doctors are compelled to question their own behavior, to reconsider objectively many of the things that they have been taught, and to cast an eye on *prevention* rather than *intervention*, their patients inevitably enjoy beneficial results.

Many reforms have emerged in the last three or four years that constitute belated recognition by doctors that the side effects of many drugs are more dangerous than the ailments they seek to correct, that elective surgery is often unnecessary and always dangerous, and that the risks of many routine tests, x-rays, and examinations are greater than those of the diseases that they are employed to detect.

During the last few years many of medicine's most cherished procedures have come into disrepute because they could not withstand the public scrutiny to which they were being subjected. For example:

- The American Academy of Pediatrics has advised against routine administration of chest x-rays when children are admitted to hospitals, a tacit acknowledgment of the potential cumulative hazards of radiology.

- The Academy has also reversed its position on routine use of the tuberculin test, except in areas of high incidence of the disease. Hopefully, this may be the first step toward elimination of all dangerous and unnecessary screening tests and immunizations that benefit the doctors who administer them more than their patients.

- The routine annual physical examination has been scrapped by the American Medical Association.

- The American Cancer Society (ACS) no longer recommends routine annual Pap smears and, for a time, also stopped recommending routine periodic mammographies. Although no convincing new evidence has emerged to support the decision—other than the outcry of underemployed radiologists—the ACS has reversed its position again. It now maintains that a mammography every one or two years is a safe and highly recommended practice for symptomless women, ages 40 to 50. This is in contradiction of the guidelines set by the National Cancer Institute in 1977, which restrict X-rays screening in this age group to women with a personal or family history of breast cancer. In my view, annual mammographies for symptom-free women are a form of self-fulfilling diagnosis. Perform enough of them and they may produce the breast cancer they are used to detect!

- Routine chest X-rays, once considered so essential that mobile units provided access to them, have gone by the boards.

- Although the pharmaceutical companies keep churning out new drugs, there is increasing patient resistance to overmedication, and fewer drugs are being prescribed. The number of prescriptions filled in 1980 was *100 million* fewer than in 1974. Perhaps as a consequence, the drug industry is putting enormous pressure on the Food and Drug Administration to permit it to advertise prescription drugs to *consumers*, not just to doctors.

- Tranquilizer prescriptions dropped from 104.5 million in 1973 to 70.8 million in 1981. The use of Valium—a major source of drug overdose fatalities—has been cut in half from a peak of 62 million prescriptions in 1975.

- Sleeping pill prescriptions dropped from a high of 40 million to 21 million in 1980.

- Increasing numbers of women are rejecting the Pill and intrauterine birth control devices because of the hazards they present.

- Breastfeeding is on the rise—a boon to both mothers and babies—despite the continuing failure of many obstetricians and pediatricians to encourage it with vigor.

- Obstetrical procedures are being questioned and modified, and there is a slow but gradual movement toward natural childbirth and even home birth.

These remarkable alterations of cherished medical practices and procedures make it clear that the profession *is* responding to a rising chorus of criticism. Not so, however, in my own specialty—pediatrics—which has emerged relatively unscathed and unaltered until now. In the pages that follow I will expose pediatric practice to the same critical scrutiny that I devoted to other segments of the medical profession in earlier books. But because pediatrics *is* my specialty, which I have practiced and taught for more than a quarter-century, I feel competent to do more than point out its flaws. This book will offer appropriate advice to parents who want to avoid the risk and expense of needless intervention while providing the care that will assure the health of their children. (For literary convenience—yours and mine—the pronoun *he* will be used throughout this book to refer to both boys and girls.)

Without attempting to be encyclopedic, I will offer specific advice on the medical problems that your child is likely to encounter from the moment of conception to the day he leaves the nest. You will learn how to tell when he is seriously ill, how you can deal with problems that don't require medical attention, how to determine when you should call your doctor, and how to assure that the treatments prescribed for your children are appropriate and safe.

With this basic information all parents can assume a larger role in maintaining the health of their children. However, this does not mean that you should assume the doctor's role, doing badly those things that a good doctor can do well. Despite the deficiencies of medical schools, doctors *do* learn technical skills that parents should not try to perform. This book will teach you what you need to know to care for most of the ills that may afflict your child, but also how to know when prudence demands that you employ a doctor's skills.

If you read the chapters that follow carefully, they will resolve most of your doubts and fears about the health of your child and help you prepare him or her for a long, healthy, and happy life!

Robert S. Mendelsohn, M.D.
Evanston, Illinois

1

Most Things Get Better by Morning

This book was written for parents who are seeking advice on how to raise healthy children, parents who are eager to give their kids a good start in life without entrusting all of the medical decisions to their pediatricians. My purpose is to help you determine when your child needs medical attention and when medical intervention should be avoided because it may do more harm than good. I also intend to alert you to the hazards of drugs, tests, X-rays, and other treatments that your pediatrician may want to employ—forms of medical intervention that may actually inflict damage on your child.

Pediatricians enjoy one significant advantage over other medical specialists because they can exploit the wholesome tendency of most parents to be more concerned about the health of their children than about their own health. Think about that for a moment. If you awaken at night with a splitting headache, what do you do? If you are like most adults, you probably get up, take an aspirin, and go back to bed. Very likely you soon fall asleep and feel fine when you wake up in the morning.

Now consider how you react when your child awakens in the middle of the night with the same symptom. Your first impulse may well be to talk to your pediatrician as soon as you can get him on the phone.

If you reach the doctor instead of his answering service, his response is predictable. Chances are he'll ask, "Did you take his temperature?" Then, whatever your response, "Well, I don't think it is anything to worry about. Give him an aspirin and bring him to the office in the morning." You hang up the phone, regretting that you made the call, give Jimmy the aspirin, and he soon goes back to sleep. So do you. You are relieved when Jimmy awakens in the morning, eagerly demanding his breakfast, and chipper as can be. After he's been fed, you wonder whether to take him to the doctor or ignore that request and spare yourself the effort and expense.

That's the way that scene is usually played, and it's a bad scene that parents should avoid. With a simple head-ache as the only symptom, there was no need to call the doctor, and even less reason to see him in the morning. Unless your child displays evidence of serious illness, a visit to his pediatrician will yield no benefit but may invite needless medical interventions that could make a well child sick!

If you have read other books on child health, you will appreciate that this is an unconventional view. Most of those books are written by doctors, and even those that honestly acknowledge the self-limiting nature of most childhood ailments are consistent with all the others in one respect. Whatever the symptom or ailment, "See your doctor" is the bottom line. The thesis of this book, predicated on nearly three decades of pediatric teaching and practice, is not "See your doctor." That may surprise you, but what I have learned during those years is that the vast majority of childhood illnesses do not require medical attention and that, when they receive it needlessly, the treatment given may do more harm than good. Consequently, my advice to parents, based on long observation of the behavior of other doctors, and my own experience in treating thousands of children, is "Avoid your doctor whenever you can."

Let me share with you some other premises that form the basis for that advice and the recommendations that I will make in the pages that follow:

- At least 95 percent of the ailments that children are prey to *will heal themselves* and do not require medical attention.

- Too often, the risk of careless or needless medical intervention is greater than the dangers of the illness itself.

- Pediatricians spend most of their time treating parental distress. The child rarely needs treatment but gets it anyway and is subjected to the consequences, and it is the parent who gets the relief. That's because most doctors believe that parents demand, or at least expect, that they will do something for the child. What concerned parents really need is reassurance, and what their kids don't need is treatment when they aren't really sick. Most doctors won't take the time to provide meaningful parental reassurance; it is quicker and easier to write a prescription for the child.

- Mother Nature, mothers, grandmothers—yes, even fathers and grandfathers—are the best doctors around, because they do not share the typical doctor's compulsion to interfere with the body's efforts and ability to heal itself.

- At least 90 percent of the drugs prescribed by pediatricians are unnecessary and a costly risk to the child who takes them. All drugs are toxic and thus dangerous, per se. Beyond that, excessive childhood use of prescription drugs may generate the belief that there is "a pill for every ill." This may lead the child to seek chemical solutions to emotional problems later in life.

- At least 90 percent of children's surgery is unnecessary, needlessly exposing the patient to the risks of death from the surgery itself, from anesthesia, or from infections contracted in the hospital, which is an inescapably germ-ridden environment.

- Most pediatricians have received little or no education covering the fundamentals of nutrition and pharmacology, and no emphasis is placed on these vital subjects in medical school. Their patients suffer because of the pediatricians' ignorance of the impact of diet on health and of the hazards and side effects of the drugs he prescribes.

- Parents need to learn when to call a doctor, and what they can do, without a doctor's intervention, to reinforce the body's ability to heal itself.

I realize that I would be placing an unfair burden on you, as a parent, if I simply described the shortcomings of pediatric practice and urged you to avoid doctors and assume greater responsibility for your children's health. It is one thing for you to accept that kind of advice when your own health is involved and quite another to accept it when you are making medical decisions in behalf of a beloved child.

This understandable ambivalence places parents at the mercy of their pediatricians. Most of the children seen by pediatricians require no treatment, but they often get it anyway. Your child's doctor has strong incentives to make you feel better by treating your child. That behavior does not square with my ethical precepts, but in practice the pediatrician who employs it is rewarded financially and psychologically for "curing" a child who wasn't seriously ill.

The financial incentives derive from the fact that a dwindling number of patients and an increasing oversupply of pediatricians are combining to curtail the income that pediatric practices generate. In order to stabilize his annual income, the doctor has an incentive to intervene more aggressively, performing questionable tests and treatments, so that he can extract increased fees from each patient he treats. This incentive will undoubtedly grow in the years ahead, as the oversupply of pediatricians becomes an even larger problem for the doctors in this field.

The psychological incentive stems from the pediatrician's need to feel that he is doing something productive. That's not easy for him to do when most of the patients he sees don't really need his skills.

Surveys of pediatricians have shown that many do not find their work rewarding; as many as one-third indicate that they are seriously considering changing their career direction to obtain "greater challenge" or because they feel "burned out." For some, the temptation to display their knowledge and thus win the gratitude of parents, even when the treatment is superfluous and even potentially damaging, can be overwhelming.

This indefensible medical behavior is a real threat to your child. You need to be constantly alert to the deficiencies of pediatric practice so that you can monitor the behavior of your child's doctor and avoid hazardous treatment that he doesn't need. But simply knowing what's wrong with pediatricians isn't much help when your child has a headache, or a pain in the belly, or a racking cough—and a fever, to boot. You need the ability to identify the conditions that require medical attention and distinguish them from those that will most likely cure themselves. Most parents also need to know more about the treatments to avoid or even reject because they are inappropriate and potentially harmful to their children.

Because most childhood illnesses respond to normal bodily defenses that may be impeded by medical treatment, use of your natural skills is usually preferable to those of a doctor in giving your child the help he needs. Moreover you will play the principal role in helping your child *avoid* illnesses by providing the wholesome nutrition that he needs and by making certain that he avoids the foods he shouldn't have. This book is intended to help you by providing the information you need to sharpen your skills and give you confidence as you raise your healthy child.

2

Parents *and* Grandparents Are Wiser than Doctors

Parents often believe I'm joking when I tell them that mothers, fathers, and grandparents are more capable than doctors of managing the health of children. Yet I firmly believe it, for reasons that are at once simple and profound.

Unless you have passed the half-century mark and were brought up outside the major cities of our country, you can't be expected to remember the classic "family doctor," for today there are scarcely any to be found. Those of us who can remember them are apt to do so with feelings of warmth and affection, for we recall the family doctor as a friendly, sensitive, unpretentious, reassuring, compassionate figure in our lives.

The family doctor of that era often had been intimately involved with our families for two, three, and even four generations. He knew each of us as individual personalities, was sensitive to our attitudes, moods, and idiosyncrasies. He viewed us as human beings in need of help, not as clinical subjects for all of the technological and pharmacological interventions that doctors today have substituted for careful examination and common sense.

Our family doctor knew our medical histories and often those of our parents and grandparents as well.

Most of the time he listened to us without impatience, answered our questions thoughtfully, calmed our fears, and explained simply and clearly what was going on in our bodies and our minds. His office was warm, comfortable, and nonthreatening, and he had a personality to match it. If we felt too sick to go there, he came to us, believing that it made more sense for a healthy doctor to visit a sick patient than vice versa. He didn't let his medical education and his ego get in the way of his humanity and his common sense. If we needed a pill, we got one, but more often he allayed our fears and anxieties with nothing more than calm reassurance and a friendly pat on the head and let nature do its work without interference.

I'll confess that in my mind's eye this appealing ghost may be somewhat romanticized, but even allowing for that, what he was is what today's doctors should be. Unfortunately, few of them are, so it falls to you, the parent, to assume that role in maintaining the health of your child.

How can I assert that parents, with no medical training, are better able than pediatricians to meet most of the health needs of their children? Simply because you are willing and able to give your children time and attention, and your doctor is not. The most important elements in the diagnosis of illness are behavior change, appearance, and the medical history of the child. As the parent, you are extremely sensitive to your child's behavior patterns, quick to note a change in his or her appearance, and totally familiar with the child's medical history, your own, and probably those of your parents as well. The typical pediatrician, whose assembly line spews out 30, 40, or even 50 patients a day, doesn't know your child as you do and has neither the time nor the inclination to learn. All of his technology—his tests and shots and x-rays and drugs and theory—in *most* instances are no substitute for the commonsense care that you, as an informed parent, can provide.

That's why your pediatrician can never be the primary authority on whether your child is sick and why you should never let him be. You are far better qualified to judge the physical condition of your child than your doctor is, simply because you know the child better. You live with your kids and observe their behavior and appearance with interest and concern, day by day.

GUIDELINES FOR DIAGNOSIS

If your child doesn't feel sick, look sick, and act sick, the odds are that he isn't sick, or certainly not sick enough to require medical attention. How many times have you been tempted to call the doctor when your child complained of a stomachache or headache and then were glad that you didn't when you found him roughhousing with his brothers and sisters within an hour or two?

I have just given you the first of three rules that you can use to guide you in diagnosis, but I'll repeat it because it is the most important:

Rule No. 1: *If your child doesn't feel sick, look sick, and act sick, he probably isn't sick.*

Rule No. 2: *Give Mother Nature ample time to work her magic before you expose your child to the potential physical and emotional side effects of treatments that your doctor may administer.* The human body has a remarkable capacity to heal itself—a capacity that in most cases surpasses anything that medical science can do—and it doesn't produce unwanted side effects.

Rule No. 3: *Common sense is the most useful tool in dealing with illness. Your doctor is less likely to employ it than you are, and certainly no more able,* *because that's not what they taught him in medical school!*

Granted, there are infrequent illnesses of critical nature for which competent medical treatment is essential, but in the case of children they are the exception rather than the rule. The obvious question is "How can parents tell which ones are serious and which are not?"

The answer is that you can't always tell, and for that matter, neither can your doctor. However, when you have finished reading this book you will be able to determine the seriousness of most of your child's ailments and will need to consult a doctor only in the limited number of instances when you are in doubt.

I have observed, in both the teaching and the practice of medicine, that most doctors do a competent job of treating patients who are very sick and a miserable job of caring for those who are well. This is the major flaw in medical education. The medical student and the pediatric resident, for that matter, learn precious little about how to keep children well, because their education begins with the premise that everyone who comes to their office will require treatment.

In medical school the student gets about three months of pediatric instruction, devoted largely to the discussion of childhood diseases that had importance decades ago when the curriculum was written but now have virtually disappeared. He absorbs a lot of biased information about immunizations but is taught very little about pharmacology, despite the fact that as a practicing physician he'll hook more kids on drugs than the most diligent pusher in town.

Only about 60 hours are devoted specifically to pharmacology during four years in the typical medical school, and most of that time is spent absorbing irrelevant information about abstract pharmacological theory. Ultimately, most of what doctors know about the drugs they administer to their patients is taught them by an army of pharmaceutical salesmen/promoters euphemistically known as "detail men." If you were to equate this relationship to the distribution of street drugs, the detail man would be the supplier and the doctor the pusher.

DOCTORS AREN'T TAUGHT THE IMPORTANCE OF NUTRITION

Virtually nothing is done in medical school to teach students that nutrition may often be the most important element of diagnosis and treatment. Consequently, they begin their practice unaware that food allergies are the primary cause of many childhood ailments and that adequate nutrition is the basis of good health. This ignorance compels them to use drugs in the treatment of diseases that could have been cured with a simple change in diet.

If the medical student has the opportunity to get some brief hands-on experience in a well-baby clinic, he won't learn very much about the real world of medicine he is soon to enter. Virtually all of his time will be spent administering immunizations, dispensing vitamins, and passing out samples of infant formula supplied by the manufacturer's detail man. The patients he sees have come to the clinic for routine, periodic physical examinations, so he'll rarely see a patient who is really sick and isn't taught how to recognize one who is.

Fledgling doctors are taught to scoff at the holistic health practitioners, at nutritional therapy, and at any other form of health care that does not require an M.D. They learn to rail at "quackery," yet no one points out to them the abundance of quackery that exists within conventional medicine itself. How can any doctor rationalize condemning those who treat patients with Laetrile when he has been guilty of feeding his own patients Bendectin, Oraflex, Zomax, or thalidomide, until they were removed from the market because of the damage attributed to them?

What little doctors learn about breastfeeding, the most effective long-term health protection a child can obtain, is usually taught by male doctors who, for obvious reasons, have little interest or experience in this vital function. Despite its enormous influence on the development and ultimate health of your baby, which I will discuss later, I heard only one lecture on breastfeeding during four years in medical school. But the formula makers were wide awake while my instructors slept, and I was brainwashed by a deluge of literature that *they* supplied.

What students *do* learn in medical school seems to relate as much to succeeding in business as to keeping their patients well. They are taught to *behave* like doctors, to project the appearance and demeanor of omnipotence, so their patients will hold them in awe.

You may assume that the inadequacies of medical school are overcome during the pediatric residency, but they're not. There the resident deals with hospitalized patients and learns to use cannon to fend off mosquitoes because of the emphasis on hazardous diagnostic technology, surgery, and other drastic procedures that are typical of the hospital routine. He still gets little or no experience in dealing with the vast majority of childhood illnesses that are brought to a pediatrician for care.

That translates, in private practice, to a compulsion to overreact to simple illnesses with dramatic forms of intervention; it is a hazard that demands your constant vigilance. I'll be more specific about that throughout this book.

When he completes his residency and opens his first office, the typical pediatrician is poorly educated and largely unskilled. He knows very little about the risks of the drastic treatments he administers, the side effects of the drugs he prescribes, the risks of the surgery he orders or performs, the possible inaccuracy of the tests on which he relies, or the shortcomings of the medical technology he employs. He knows virtually nothing about the most critical items in pediatric health care—the impact of nutritional, allergic, psychological, and emotional factors on the well-being of his patients.

Pediatricians actually spend most of their time treating patients who don't need treatment and refer to specialists most of those who are injured or seriously ill. In fact, the referral of patients to other specialists is such an intergral part of their function that they are sometimes referred to as "access managers" within the medical profession.

Perhaps because I've been a pediatrician for so long, I have little remaining conviction that a specialist is needed to perform this function. Most childhood illnesses can be treated competently within the home, by informed and caring parents. When medical treatment is indicated it can be provided as well by general practitioners or family practitioners or by specialists to whom their patients are referred. In fact, given the opportunity, nurse-practitioners could perform most of these functions equally well. That is actually the practice in many other countries that have only a relative handful of pediatricians yet produce medical outcomes that are better than ours.

It may seem anomalous, but those outcomes are better *because* there are fewer pediatricians. Children in those countries are healthier because there is less medical intervention and thus less exposure to potentially damaging drugs and medical technology. Although American medical schools teach their students very little about pharmacology, they do teach them to exploit all of the new drugs and medical technologies that are available. New drugs and equipment appear almost daily, spawned by the laboratories of the pharmaceutical industry and the medical equipment manufacturers. More often than not, they are unproven and potentially unsafe.

Most parents assume, as they should have the right

to, that they can rely on the federal Food and Drug Administration to keep drugs off the market until they have been proven safe for human use. Most doctors, who *don't* have the right to because they know better, operate on that premise, too. This confidence in the FDA is misplaced, because virtually all drugs are released without appropriate or significant human trials. They may have immediate or short-term effects of some patients that have not been discovered. Even more likely is the possibility of cumulative and long-term effects, which I will discuss more fully in a later chapter. These long-term effects are *never* known at the time new drugs are introduced and perhaps not for decades after that, when untold harm has already been done to unsuspecting victims.

The history of medicine, here and abroad, is replete with examples of drugs approved for human use that were removed from the market only after countless victims bore evidence of the damage they caused. You may recall some of the more sensational examples—DES, MER 29, thalidomide. To compound the problem, although the FDA has the power to keep unproven drugs off the market, it has virtually no authority to force their removal once they have been approved. It also lacks an effective postmarketing surveillance mechanism that would alert it and the public to the appearance of destructive effects from the drugs that have been released. That's why the hazards of drugs are most often publicly revealed in European nations, which do exercise postmarketing surveillance that brings their risks to light.

DOCTORS RARELY INVESTIGATE THE DRUGS THEY USE

It is a rare doctor, indeed, who investigates the tests to which a drug or a treatment has been subjected before he begins to use it on his patients. Even when doubts are raised about commonly prescribed drugs, most doctors pay no attention to them. The manufacturers of several of the drugs doctors most frequently prescribe for children have been ordered by the FDA to offer proof that they are safe and effective or remove them from the market. The manufacturers have been sparring with the FDA for years, while still selling these drugs. In most instances they have yet to come up with proof that these drugs are any good, yet doctors keep right on prescribing them. I'm not talking about a handful of drugs but—literally—hundreds of them.

It seems almost incredible, but American parents spend millions of dollars every year on drugs that their doctors have prescribed without any evidence that the drugs are effective or safe or, worse, in the face of responsible allegations that they are not. Of the 30 drugs labeled ineffective by the FDA that were most frequently prescribed in 1979, more than half—including the top three—are often prescribed for children. Those on the list include Dimetapp, Actifed, Donnatal, Ornade Spansules, Phenergan Expectorant, Tuss-Ornade, Phenergan VC Expectorant with Codeine, Actifed C Expectorant, Bentyl, Phenergan Expectorant Plain, Benylin Cough Syrup, Marax and Marax DF, Dimetane Expectorant, Ambenyl Expectorant, Dimetane Expectorant DC, and Teldrin. Next time your doctor prescribes one of them for your child, ask him why he is using a drug that the manufacturer has been unable to defend as doing any good.

During the early years of my practice, when I was still naive enough to believe what they had taught me in medical school, I was guilty of the same sort of behavior. During my pediatric residency I was taught to use x-rays to treat the tonsils, acne, ringworm of the scalp, and enlarged lymph and thymus glands. No one told me that I need to have any concern about the long-term consequences of this treatment, nor did it occur to me to question whether I might be causing my patients future harm.

In those days I took everything on faith and expected my patients to do likewise. I'm ashamed of that now and suspicious of every new medical fad, because those x-ray treatments were responsible for a virtual epidemic of thyroid cancer among patients subjected to them. The damage that was done is still being discovered every day. Even more tragic is the fact that in the case of enlarged lymph and thymus glands, we were treating nonailments. Their size ultimately diminished without treatment, in the natural order of things.

Who knows what the future consequences will be of the things pediatric residents are being taught today? They are learning to use bilirubin lights to treat infant jaundice, tympanostomy for ear infections, antibiotics for almost everything, hormones to control growth, powerful drugs to modify child behavior, and other drugs, tests, immunizations, and procedures whose long-term effects are unknown. The consequences have yet to be fully revealed, but if you reexamine the previous disasters that litter the path of "medical progress" you can be sure they will be many and tragic.

If there is a given about medical practice, it is that doctors don't seem to learn anything from their mistakes and that most of them seem oblivious to the basic tenet of the Hippocratic oath, "First, do no harm." Doctors do a lot of harm, but the very structure of their medical education over time makes them insensitive to the harm that they do.

"We want our doctors to be caring and sensitive," Daniel Borenstein, of the UCLA School of Medicine, said recently, "but if they are overly caring, it's difficult for them to continue to function. Throughout medical school there's a hardening of the spirit."

The pediatric resident may become quite skilled in certain mechanical procedures frequently performed in hospitals, such as inserting needles into veins and arteries, performing spinal taps, and even inserting tracheal and bronchial tubes. However, these skills diminish rapidly after he leaves the hospital and stops using them. Within a year or two, you can't depend on him to retain many of the skills he learned. Fortunately for him, and for his patients, it doesn't make much difference because he rarely needs to use them. They were typically learned while treating children in pediatric clinics who were the victims of economic deprivation, inadequate hygiene, and poor nutrition and consequently suffered ailments rarely seen in middle-class or affluent pediatric practices. Since most pediatricians go where the money is, there isn't much chance that they'll continue to treat poor children when they enter private practice. In fact, most of the time they'll be treating kids who don't need treatment because they aren't seriously ill.

WHAT DOCTORS ARE TAUGHT TO DO ABOUT MISTAKES

As part of my preparation for entering private practice I was taught during my pediatric residency what to do if I made a terrible mistake. I wasn't told what to tell the parents of the child so that they could handle their grief more adequately, nor was I given any ethical standards to adhere to. Instead, I was admonished to call my malpractice insurance carrier immediately and let him tell me how to proceed. If I had to say anything publicly about a grievous—perhaps fatal—error, the magic phrase was, "What happened to this poor child was one in a million."

That's why, when something goes wrong, you'll often hear a doctor say, "It was one in a million." In Toronto there was the famous case of Stephen Yuz, who entered the Hospital for Sick Children and was diagnosed as having psychological vomiting. He died some days later from an intestinal obstruction. It was one in a million, of course, as was the death of a Chicago child as the result of an asthma test.

I have attempted, in this chapter, to dissuade you from having blind faith in your pediatrician and to point out that when you seek medical attention that your child doesn't really need you may expose him to greater risks. Medical attention should be your last resort—not your first—when your child is sick. The vast majority of childhood illnesses will respond to natural bodily defenses, fortified by your own skills, loving attention, and common sense.

How Doctors
Can Make
Healthy Kids Sick

If you think about the relationships you have had with doctors, I suspect you'll be surprised to discover that they're unlike those you have with anyone else who provides you with a service. The typical doctor-patient relationship is revealed in a phrase that has become part of the language, *doctor's orders*. Doctors *do* give *give orders* to their patients; lawyers, accountants, and other professionals give *advice*.

When you take your child to a pediatrician he conducts a physical examination that is too often cursory rather than thorough; orders tests and x-rays; makes a diagnosis; decides on a course of treatment, often requiring drugs; and sometimes admits him to a hospital for an extended stay. He does all this with a minimum of explanation, without asking for your approval, usually without warning you about the risks and potential side effects of the treatment he is giving, and without telling you what it is all going to cost. When it is all over he will expect you to pay your bill, even if the diagnosis was wrong, or the treatment didn't work, and your child is still sick. Doctors, in short, have minimal accountability to their patients for anything they do.

Americans clearly are at the mercy of their doctors, and as a parent you are even more so because your concern for a child who can't make his own decisions makes you particularly vulnerable. Your child, in turn, becomes vulnerable to treatment that is often painful and debilitating. Because doctors are taught in medical school to submerge any emotional response to human suffering, they simply don't pay enough attention to the pain they inflict and the damage that their treatments may cause.

Among doctors as a group, I believe the pediatrician is the most dangerous because he appears to be the most benign. The image of a pediatrician is most often that of a smiling, kindly, caring professional who, along with his prescriptions, gives balloons and lollipops to your kids. He undeservedly escapes the opprobrium that is sometimes directed toward obstetricians and surgeons, who are more likely to be viewed as callous and money-grubbing.

WHY PEDIATRICIANS ARE DANGEROUS

The confidence inspired by the demeanor of pediatricians is, in my experience, undeserved. It tends to mask the elements of pediatric practice that are threatening to your child. Let me recite briefly some of the reasons why I believe pediatricians are dangerous and then get into the most serious of them later, in greater detail.

1. The pediatrician serves as the recruiter for the medical profession. He indoctrinates your child from birth into a lifelong dependence on medical intervention. It begins with a succession of needless "well-baby checkups" and immunizations and then moves on to routine annual physical examinations and endless treatment of minor ailments that would cure themselves if they were left alone.

2. Pediatricians are the least likely of all specialists to tell parents about the potential side effects of the drugs and treatments they prescribe. What pediatrician ever told mothers of the evidence linking infant formula to high blood lead levels and Sudden Infant Death Syn-

drome (SIDS)? What pediatrician, until pressured to do so by media revelations, ever told parents of the risk of epilepsy and mental retardation associated with the immunizations that he performs? What pediatrician tells parents that antibiotics should be reserved for cases in which there is no acceptable option, that frequent and indiscriminate use may have adverse future consequences for the child?

3. The pediatrician's wanton prescribing of powerful drugs indoctrinates children from birth with the philosophy of "a pill for every ill." This may lead the child to the belief that there is a drug to treat every condition and that drugs are an appropriate response to normal feelings of frustration, depression, anxiety, inadequacy, insecurity, etc. Doctors are *directly* responsible for hooking millions of people on prescription drugs. They are also *indirectly* responsible for the plight of millions more who turn to illegal drugs because they were taught at an early age that drugs can cure anything—including psychological and emotional conditions—that ails them.

4. Pediatrics is among the lowest-paid of the medical specialties. Consequently, because he has greater need for the income they generate, the pediatrician is more likely than other doctors to order unnecessary x-rays and tests. The risks to the patient are twofold: first, potentially harmful effects from the tests and the x-rays themselves; second, the danger that inappropriate treatment may be given because the pediatrician discounted clinical evidence in making his diagnosis and relied on test results that too often are unreliable.

5. Pediatricians are so accustomed to seeing patients who aren't really sick that they often fail to recognize the ones who are. I have been an expert witness in many malpractice suits that bear this out. Board-certified pediatricians have overlooked important, life-threatening conditions because they had forgotten what to look for in a sick child and missed the symptoms that should have alerted them to a serious condition.

Meningitis is an outstanding example of this shortcoming, because it is today one of the rarities in pediatrics. It used to be 95-percent fatal and now is 95-percent curable, but only if the pediatrician recognizes the symptoms and identifies the disease in time. Every pediatrician, during his residency, is taught how to diagnose meningitis. In fact, it is one of the few really useful things that he is taught. But that lesson is often blotted out after years of examining a procession of healthy children. To make matters worse, the pediatrician gets so accustomed to treating nonailments that when he does properly diagnose a sick child he may no longer remember the appropriate treatment.

6. Because they see more children in order to enjoy a profitable practice, pediatricians don't spend enough time with their patients to diagnose and treat them properly. Every competent physician knows that 85 percent of an accurate diagnosis is based on the patient's history, 10 percent on a thorough physical examination, and the remainder on laboratory tests and x-rays. It takes at least half an hour to an hour to take an adequate history and to conduct a thorough physical exam. Pediatricians typically spend 10 minutes with a patient and thus fail to discern much of what they need to know for a reliable diagnosis because they simply don't spend the time that is needed. The result is "knee jerk" or "cookie cutter" diagnosis, in which habit replaces sound judgment based on careful examination.

7. Pediatricians are the most likely of all specialists to enhance their income by promoting and defending laws that force patients to use their services. It is pediatricians, not politicians, who are responsible for mandatory use of silver nitrate or antibiotic drops in a newborn's eyes, mandatory school physical examinations that provide opportunities for "creative diagnosis" of nonailments, mandatory hospital births, and court-ordered use of controversial and unproven methods of treatment to which the parents object. Increasingly, one of the dangers inherent in taking your child to the doctor is the possibility that he may be taken from you and placed in

state custody if you reject the treatment that his doctor demands. I have testified in behalf of the parents in many such legal actions in recent years.

8. Pediatricians are the principal foes of breastfeeding, despite incontrovertible evidence that it is one of the most effective ways to assure the future health of your child. Although the LaLeche League is beginning to counter the influence that the formula makers have long had on pediatricians, many doctors either fail to encourage or actively discourage breastfeeding. I won't go into all of the reasons for this, but it is worth noting that the growth of the pediatric specialty in the United States can be attributed in large measure to the financial support of the manufacturers of infant formula, who have long used pediatricians as unpaid salesmen.

9. Pediatricians give tacit support to the unconscionable obstetrical intervention that is damaging children, physically and intellectually. They cover up the obstetricians' role in producing much of the damage that they see. When a parent has a child with a birth defect, and asks a pediatrician whether the obstetrician might be responsible, he will get the reply that is taught during pediatric residency: "Don't look back; just look ahead." Dangerous obstetrical practices that produce retardation, learning disabilities, and physical abnormalities would disappear in a few years if pediatricians had the courage and compassion to place the blame on obstetricians, which is often where it belongs.

Despite all this evidence of negative effects from pediatric care, the myth persists that American children enjoy better health care because of our abundance of pediatricians. That belief is wrong on two counts. First, infant mortality statistics reveal that American children are less healthy than those in many other developed nations that have few pediatricians. They're even less healthy than children in some of the underdeveloped countries. Second, the reason our children are less healthy may well be *because* of our abundance of pediatricians.

Despite evidence to the contrary, public health policy in the United States is based on the premise that access to care determines the health of a population. Doctors have succeeded in convincing politicians of this, even though they can't prove it. I believe that as long as emergency medical services are available, access to *routine* medical care probably has a negative effect on health. We've seen it happen in California, Saskatchewan, Israel, and elsewhere: *call a doctor's strike and the death rate goes down*!

KEY TO HEALTH: STAY AWAY FROM DOCTORS!

The best way to raise a healthy child is to keep him away from doctors, except for emergency care in the case of an accident or an obviously serious illness. If your child displays symptoms of illness, monitor his condition closely, but don't seek medical help until there are clear indications that he is seriously ill. Most doctors ignore the fact that the human body is a wondrous machine with an astonishing capacity to repair itself. If you take your sick child to a doctor, he probably won't allow it to do that. Instead, he will interfere with the body's natural defenses by giving your child treatment that he doesn't need and shouldn't get, with side effects that his body is not designed to handle.

If you become convinced that you should accept my advice and avoid your doctor whenever it makes sense to do so, you will learn to avoid the traps that pediatric medicine has laid for your child. The first of these is the "well-baby visit"—a cherished ritual of pediatricians that enhances their income but does nothing constructive for your child. The hazard of these examinations is the proclivity of doctors—a heritage of medical school—to discover illness where none exists. The diagnosis leads to treatment, of course, with consequences that may make your child sick.

The time to see a doctor is when your child is really sick, not when he's well. If your pediatrician asks that you bring your baby in for routine, regular checkups on a monthly, bimonthly, or other regularly scheduled basis, ask him why he thinks this is necessary. Ask him if he knows of any objective studies that indicate it will have any effect in improving your child's health. I've never seen one, and I don't believe he will be able to point to one, either.

Although professional groups have recommended that the value of preventive child health care be validated by conducting controlled studies that follow patients over many years, little research has been done. The three studies that I have seen offered no support to pediatricians who demand that their patients visit them on a regular basis. The studies focused individually on general health, behavioral patterns and learning abilities, and developmental status, as the end points of the research. As reported in *Pediatrics*, "None of these studies provided evidence that the preventive services given affected the outcomes measured positively."

In the absence of any evidence that well-baby visits will improve the health of your child, I suggest you avoid them and the risks of needless treatment they present and save your time and money. In all my years as a pediatrician *I do not recall ever having discovered an illness during a well-baby examination that was not revealed in a timely manner by taking a careful history on the child's initial visit or by the subsequent development of observable symptoms*. I'll discuss that more fully later.

Well-baby visits are worthless because they are essentially superficial, and they are superficial because the doctor knows deep in his heart, that they are a waste of time. Another study conducted in metropolitan Pittsburgh revealed that pediatricians conduct a well-baby visit in an average of a little more than 10 minutes and then provide advice on child development, potential problems, and similar matters in an average of *52 seconds*. Similar findings were reported in New York City, Baltimore, Seattle, Los Angeles, and Rochester, New York.

No doctor can diagnose a symptom-free disease in 10 minutes or give any constructive advice in 52 seconds. If my child were the patient, I wouldn't even give a doctor the opportunity to try.

When your child enters a pediatric examining room he is almost invariably subjected to height and weight measurements, usually taken by a technician or a nurse. This is part of the ritual Modern Medicine has developed to make you feel that you are getting your money's worth. First-time parents wait nervously while the nurse places the squirming baby on the scale and may be asked to help hold the child's legs down so that the height can be measured. Mom and Dad sigh with relief when their pediatrician finally appears, checks the measurements against a chart, and announces that their child is developing "normally." Conversely, they are worried if they are told that their baby is gaining too much or too little weight.

What their doctor doesn't tell them is that this ritual has no medical significance whatsoever. They aren't told that some formula manufacturer was probably the source of the growth chart that the doctor is using and that he gets them free. That leads to an obvious question: Why are the formula makers so eager to have your doctor check your baby's weight? Answer: Because the weight gain of breastfed babies may not match the average weights shown on the formula maker's chart. They hope that the pediatrician, instead of reassuring the mother that this is normal and nonthreatening, will tell her to stop breastfeeding and switch to their product, of which he has a handy reminder in his hand. Too often, that is exactly what he does, and the baby is subsequently denied the immunity and other benefits that breastfeeding provides.

For at least half a century doctors have been relying

on various standard weight and height tables to measure the health of patients of all ages. For older children and adults the most commonly used chart is one developed by the Metropolitan Life Insurance Company, last revised in 1959. The pediatrician compares your child's height and weight measurements to those on the average growth curve. If the child is at either end of the spectrum, he will be defined as "abnormal." The doctor misleads the parent by evaluating a single patient on the basis of a theoretical statistical value.

WHY WEIGHT CHARTS ARE MISLEADING

This evaluation is misleading because the charts are based on an average of a group of subjects that may not be comparable—environmentally, racially, or genetically—to your child. The doctor makes the assumption that, unless your child is near the 50th percentile, he is either too skinny or too fat, too tall or too short. If the measurements are well removed from the midpoint, the doctor can then seize the opportunity to treat your child.

This indefensible practice reminds me of a definition I once heard of the role of lawyers, whose function, it was said, was "to raise doubts in the minds of their clients, which they can then resolve over a long period of time at great profit to themselves." That's what is happening when a pediatrician uses variations from "normal" height and weight as an excuse to treat your child.

Comparison of individual children to charts of average height and weight is unscientific, per se, and becomes more so when you consider that the charts themselves are invalid. As this is written there is a raging debate over the Metropolitan Life charts, which many doctors have challenged as defining ideal adult weights 10-20 pounds too low. It appears that Metropolitan will respond to this criticism by raising the weight standards, and another group of doctors is challenging that. Whatever the result, one thing is certain. Doctors will ignore this history and continue to compare your child to whatever standard is agreed to, as though the measurements had been handed down from a Higher Power that inscribed them on stone.

Studies have shown that the standard height and weight charts applied to children (several are in use) are even less valid than those used for adults. For example, they are meaningless when applied to measure the development of black children. That's because they are based on the progress of groups of Caucasian children, and black children exhibit different growth characteristics when studied as a group. Another deviation that the charts fail to take into account are genetic factors in child development. They make the assumption, ignoring the genetic factors, that a child with parents shorter than five feet, six inches, should attain the same height as a child whose parents are both over six feet tall.

Comparisons with standard growth charts also trouble me because no valid norms have ever been developed for breastfed babies, who often exhibit weight gains that are below those achieved by babies who are formula-fed. This is quite normal, and also beneficial, and there is no evidence that God made a mistake when he constructed breasts that don't yield Neo-Mull-Soy or Enfamil. Unfortunately, many pediatricians don't seem to believe that, so if you are breastfeeding your baby and his weight gain does not match the charts, your doctor is likely to insist on switching him to formula. That's bad for you and worse for your child. I'll have more to say on this later, but let me emphasize right now that I believe breastfeeding is a vital element in the health of children, not only in infancy but later in life.

The use of standard growth charts is an example—and American medicine is filled with them—of quantitative nonsense superseding qualitative sense. Don't let your pediatrician influence you by attaching importance to comparisons of your child's growth with any standard norms. Remember, if he tries, that these norms are based on tiny groups of children, were done many years ago, often compare apples and oranges, and don't differentiate between breastfed and bottlefed babies.

Let me repeat: Your pediatrician literally does not know the normal growth pattern of breastfed babies. He is misleading you if he tells you that your breastfed baby isn't growing fast enough. If your baby is otherwise healthy, don't switch to formula because of nonsense your pediatrician has extrapolated from his worthless charts!

I know it may be difficult for you to accept the fact that growth charts have no place in medical diagnosis, because doctors have been using them for so long. Let me assure you that I am not alone in the view that more harm than good may come from using them to measure the health and progress of an individual child. This position is shared by many other doctors who have been moved to look objectively at the results they have experienced in their own practices rather than continue to accept what they learned in medical school.

I have belabored this issue because I want it to serve as an advance warning of all the other offenses against your child that your pediatrician may commit. I'll describe many more as we move on to specific illnesses. The point is that, if a pediatrician will treat a child on the basis of information obtained from invalid charts, it is not difficult to comprehend the interventions he will conceive if he has a more tangible symptom that he can use to rationalize his behavior.

For the most part, the damage done by growth charts is limited to their impact on your pocketbook and your peace of mind. However, in recent years they have led to a major abuse that I will mention briefly only to condemn it. I refer to the growing use of estrogens and other hormones to try to alter the height of children who are perceived as being too tall or too short. Little is known about the potential damage that may be inflicted by the hormones that are being used to stimulate or retard growth, and nothing is known about the long-term effects of this treatment.

In recent years the medical journals have reported extensively on the use of estrogen to keep girls from growing "too tall." One headline, which assured readers that such treatment was "safe," noted the following risks and side effects, but they were buried deep in the text of the story: morning sickness, night cramps, thrombophlebitis (blood clots in the veins), hives, obesity, hypertension, abnormal menstrual bleeding, suppression of pituitary hormones, migraine headaches, precipitation of diabetes mellitus, gallstones, atherosclerosis, breast and genital tract cancer, and sterility. The article also noted that "relatively few girls have been treated long enough ago ... to have outlived the latent period for neoplasia [the formation of malignant tumors]."

How many doctors who recommend this treatment tell their patients about these side effects? How many parents would permit their doctor to treat a child for height control if they were made aware of the risks the treatment entails?

The risks of exposure to significant damage in the course of routine medical care are neither remote nor inconsequential. That's why you should assume the dominant role in dealing with your child's health.

4

Protecting Your
Children before
They Are Born

Most of us tend to believe that the awesome responsibility of parenting begins when we take our new baby home from the hospital. Actually many decisions that will affect the health and vitality of your child are made long before that. Your first opportunities to build a healthy foundation for your child's growth and development come before he or she is born.

While it is too late to take advantage of these opportunities if you already have your child, you should know about them anyway, in the event you plan to have another. If, however, you are reading this book in anticipation of the birth of your baby, this chapter will be of immediate importance to you.

The future well-being of your baby will be affected by choices you can make throughout your pregnancy. It can be affected by the attitudes of the obstetrician you choose. Then, when the long wait is over and the first pangs of labor appear, you may even choose to avoid the hospital and deliver your baby at home.

Please don't dismiss that choice out of hand. At first glance it may sound like radical advice, but I assure you that it isn't. A steadily increasing percentage of mothers are demanding home births for their babies, because they have examined both options and determined that home birth is the sensibly conservative choice.

What is radical—and dangerous for you and your child—is the arsenal of obstetrical intervention that lies in wait for you in the hospital, as well as the threats lurking in the hospital nursery that may damage your baby after he is born. There is ample evidence that the medical technology, drugs, anesthetics, surgery, and other obstetrical slings and arrows employed in most hospitals expose mothers and babies to needless risk. They have a frightening potential for inflicting severe, even life-threatening, damage on you and also on your child.

CHILDBIRTH SHOULD BE A NATURAL PROCESS

The classic family doctor of my own childhood "assisted" in the delivery of babies when, and to the extent that, his services were required. To him, childbirth was an uncomplicated natural process, and he did not interfere with it except in those rare instances when something went terribly wrong. If labor was prolonged, he didn't give the mother a shot of Pitocin so he could get to the golf course on time. He was content to give nature a chance and would sit with a laboring mother for hours until her body, not Parke-Davis Pharmaceutical Company, decided it was time for her to deliver.

What a contrast with the often irrational obstetrical behavior we see today! Contemporary obstetricians, for the most part, no longer "*assist*." They consistently *interfere* in a natural physiological process that they insist on treating as though it were a disease. In a shocking percentage of cases this medical interference with a normal bodily function adversely affects the physical or intellectual capacity of the child for the rest of his life. Sometimes it even ends that life before it really has a chance to begin.

If you have your baby in a hospital, you will be exposed to an array of obstetrical hazards so broad that I can't possibly describe them fully here. However, they were thoroughly documented in my previous book, *Male Practice*: *How Doctors Manipulate Women*, so if you want more information about the obstetrical risks to mothers, you will find it there. What I discuss in this and succeeding chapters are the secondary effects of obstetrical intervention on your child, and the primary damage that your doctor and the hospital's routine procedures may inflict on your baby after his birth.

Obstetricians, in defense of their own fouled nest, insist that a hospital is the only safe place for you to have your child. On occasion they even go to court to try to prevent mothers from using midwives and having their babies at home. There is no statistical or scientific evidence to defend their position; in fact, the available evidence proves them wrong. Meanwhile, observation of the iatrogenic (doctor-caused) damage to children, coupled with simple logic, is enough to demonstrate to any impartial judge that the safest place to have a baby is at home.

The reason is almost self-evident. Having your baby at home is less risky than going to the hospital because much of the most dangerous technology employed in hospitals is not available to doctors or midwives who deliver babies at home. This reduces the opportunity for needless, hazardous intervention and virtually assures that you will be permitted to have your baby naturally, as God intended that you should. Procedures such as ultrasound diagnosis, internal fetal monitoring, excessive use of sedatives, pain relievers and anesthetics, Pitocin-induced labor, and the temptation to resort to delivery by cesarean section, are largely avoided when you play it safe and have your baby in your very own bed!

Obstetricians who practice in hospitals decry home birth as reckless, because hospital facilities are not available in the event a complication arises. If those doctors, whose practice is limited to hospitals, were determining which mothers were appropriate candidates for home birth, and were then required to deal with any emergencies that arose, I would agree with them. They don't have the skill and experience to select the appropriate home birth candidates and to anticipate problems in other mothers. They also would be at a loss to cope with an occasional problem *they did not cause* and without the assistance and technology available to them in the hospital.

Home birth doctors and midwives are experienced in identifying mothers who can safely give birth at home and rejecting home birth for those who are not. They can also anticipate problems, but without the intervention that occurs in the hospital setting, these problems are few and far between, and home birth doctors know how to cope with those that do arise.

HOW BABIES ARE DAMAGED DURING HOSPITAL BIRTHS

There are five distinct stages during which you should be alert to actions of your doctors that could result in the birth of a deformed, brain-damaged, or mentally retarded child. The first is the period prior to conception; second, the nine months of pregnancy; third, while you are in labor; fourth, during the delivery of your baby; and, finally, the period during which your child remains in the hospital for newborn care. Let's examine them, and the risks they entail, one by one.

The Preconception Stage

The behavior of doctors can influence the health of your baby long before the thought of having one has even crossed your mind. The fact that you are reading this book suggests that it is too late for you to do anything about that, but it is not too late for you to take the precautions in the future that will protect your next child.

Fetal deformities and mental retardation may occur as

the result of excessive exposure to x-rays throughout your life, and these radiation effects are a threat to the health of both men and women and the children that are born to them.

Among women, the consequences of excessive exposure to radiation are usually noted among those who have their first babies in their later years. That's because the effects of X-rays are cumulative, so the older you are, the more opportunities there have been for radiation to accumulate and take its toll. This increases the possibility that Down's syndrome, a form of mental retardation, will afflict your child. Nor is this form of X-ray damage limited to women. Fathers may also be responsible for offspring with fetal deformities and mental retardation if X-ray exposure has damaged their sperm.

This potential impact on fetal development is one of many reasons why you and your children should avoid X-ray exposure to the extent that you can, from the earliest age. You can expect your doctor and dentist to downplay the risks of X-ray diagnosis, which they will maintain are minimal. Your dentist will also insist that his X-rays are harmless because the dosage is very low. Don't be misled by these assurances. It doesn't make any difference how low the dosage is during any single exposure to x-rays if you accumulate enough during your lifetime to damage you or your child.

I advise my patients to reject all X-rays unless they are essential to the diagnosis of a potentially life-threatening disease. If you must submit your child to an X-ray, don't hesitate to let your doctor know that you are concerned, even if you feel uncomfortable doing so. Your child's health is more important than your doctor's feelings. Insist that X-ray examinations be conducted at the lowest dosage possible. Ask your doctor whether his technician has been specifically trained and whether the equipment has been inspected recently to assure that it delivers the appropriate dose. Observe whether the technician provides proper shielding for the reproductive organs of your child.

Never let yourself forget that X-ray machines can be lethal. Study after study has shown that a shocking number of X-rays are performed in the United States with defective equipment, operated by untrained medical personnel who don't know how to use the machine properly. To make matters worse, most of the time the x-rays weren't essential in the first place.

You face another major risk if conception follows too closely a period of contraception with birth control pills. This, too, can result in a deformed or brain-damaged child. Women who have used the Pill should allow several months to pass before they attempt to have a child.

What to Watch for during Pregnancy

The babies who are at greatest risk during the first days, weeks, or months of life are those born prematurely, before all of their organs are fully developed, and those who lack physical stamina because of abnormally low weight at birth. You can help assure that your child will develop normally if you eat an adequate, nutritious diet from the moment of conception until the day he is born.

When I was young, doctors were fond of encouraging mothers to do this by reminding them that they were "eating for two." Today's obstetricians are more likely to be preoccupied with the insistence that you restrict your weight. Not too long ago, the maximum weight gain that many obstetricians would tolerate was 10-15 pounds. More recently, the reins your doctor will try to place on your appetite have been loosened a little, but most doctors will still try to limit your weight gain during pregnancy to 20-25 pounds. That's more rational, but the limitation still doesn't make any sense. On the contrary, maternal dietary and caloric restrictions may lower your child's birth weight and threaten his development or even his survival.

The possibility that your doctor may try to subject you to excessive weight restrictions is very real. A federal agency reported that in 1975 one of every three pregnant women in the United States suffered from malnutrition—more than a million women a year. Obviously, some of them were malnourished because they couldn't afford proper food, or for cosmetic reasons of their own, but the overwhelming majority suffered from malnutrition because their obstetricians wouldn't let them eat. Don't let your doctor do this to you, because it is virtually inevitable that, if you are malnourished, your baby will be, too.

Your primary concern during pregnancy should not be with how much weight you gain but with how adequately and well you eat. If your doctor tells you to hold your weight gain to 15-20 pounds, he will probably insist that this is important because it will make your delivery easier. He may also tell you that it will forestall the possibility that you will develop toxemia, one of the most dangerous and sometimes fatal complications of pregnancy.

These sound like persuasive reasons to control your weight, and you obviously would be wise to heed them if they were true. You needn't, because all of the available evidence indicates that in terms of ease of delivery and the threat of toxemia the truth is the other way around.

If you are malnourished, your uterus may not function properly and labor will be prolonged or even stop. The obstetrician who restricted your diet has now turned that lemon into lemonade for himself by creating the opportunity to do a cesarean section. That's a bonanza for him but potential trouble for you and your child.

And so it also is with toxemia. Evidence has been accumulating for half a century that it is improper maternal nutrition, not excess weight, that causes toxemia in pregnancy. Because the proper nutritional elements are not present in your diet, your liver malfunctions, and your body's responses produce the symptoms that are associated with toxemia.

Many women find it difficult to adhere to the weight restrictions imposed by their doctors and find themselves nearing the outer limits during the final two months of pregnancy. If they take their doctors' instructions seriously, they go on near-starvation diets, cutting down their food intake at the worst possible time. This is the period when their child needs maximum nourishment, because he should be gaining the most weight. It is also the crucial period in the development of the brain. If you starve yourself to hold to some arbitrary, medically imposed weight restriction, you also starve your baby, endangering his life and health as well as your own.

My advice to expectant mothers—no matter what their obstetricians are telling them—is to exercise common sense about food intake and how much or how fast they gain weight. But don't lose any sleep over it if you find yourself gaining more than your doctor would like. You'll feel better about it if you remember that the chances that an underweight baby will die during the first month after delivery are 30 times those of babies born at normal weight. Because they have been denied the nourishment they needed to develop properly, some degree of mental retardation is found in half of the low-birth-weight babies, and their incidence of epilepsy, cerebral palsy, and learning or behavioral problems is three times that of babies of normal weight. That's a good reason for you to eat a well-balanced, nourishing diet, avoid starving yourself or your baby, and tell your obstetrician to go fly a kite if he fusses at you because you've gained 30 pounds.

Be equally firm in your refusal if he tries to put you on diuretics should your hands and feet begin to swell. Nearly all pregnant women display swelling due to water retention at some time during pregnancy. This is almost always a normal condition and a valuable one, because the stored fluid that produces the edema is needed to support the increased blood volume that you and your baby require.

Many doctors seize this condition as an indication of toxemia and prescribe a diuretic to eliminate the stored fluids. In most cases that's wrong, because it simply de-

38

prives you and your baby of fluids you need. The result can be catastrophic. The death rate of babies born to mothers without edema has been shown to be 50 percent higher than that of babies born to mothers who stored ample fluid. You are also at risk if you take diuretics, because these drugs can kill you by lowering your blood pressure and pushing you into hypovolemic shock!

Your doctor will almost certainly warn you sternly about the hazards of cigarettes, alcohol, and other mood-altering drugs during pregnancy. He *should* warn you about them, and you should heed his warnings, because there is strong evidence that even moderate use of these substances may have a negative impact on your unborn child. For the same reason, he should also warn you not to take any over-the-counter drugs during your pregnancy—aspirin, cold remedies, and the like.

Unfortunately, he probably won't warn you about the even greater risks present in some of the treatments that he may employ. Fetal damage can also be caused by prescription drugs, x-rays taken during pregnancy, ultrasound, and procedures such as amniocentesis, which is used to detect abnormal conditions of the fetus. I won't go into these hazards here, but you should inform yourself about them. Many books about the medical hazards of pregnancy are available, including my own book, *Male Practice*: *How Doctors Manipulate Women*.

Intervention during Labor and Delivery

At the beginning of this chapter I urged you to consider home birth for your child in order to avoid the greater opportunities for medical intervention that are present if you enter a hospital. Almost every form of obstetrical intervention in what should be a natural process of birth has the potential for causing brain damage and mental retardation. The risks of such intervention, and thus the consequences, are substantially reduced if you have your baby at home.

A few years ago Dr. Lewis E. Mehl, of the University of Wisconsin infant development center, studied 2,000 births, nearly half of which had taken place at home. The differences between the home and the hospital births were striking:

- There were 30 birth injuries among the hospital-born children and none among those born at home.

- Fifty-two of the babies born in the hospital required resuscitation, against only 14 of those born at home.

- Six hospital babies suffered neurological damage, compared to one born at home.

The extent of the intervention in the birth process that typifies hospital deliveries is appalling. True, some of the procedures that are used have merit when they are appropriately applied—situations in which the risks of doing the procedure are justified by the benefits it may provide. The menace to the mother arises from the syndrome "What can be done will be done," which pervades American medicine. Procedures developed specifically to deal with critical situations are used routinely on every patient who comes in the door.

The typical hospital delivery, in most hospitals, is characterized by one needless intervention after another. Again, because I have covered them in previous books, I will not go into the details here. Included, however, are internal and external fetal monitoring, intravenous feeding, analgesics and anesthetics, Pitocin-induced labor, episiotomy, and cesarean sections.

I do want to take the opportunity here to share with you emerging information about the risks of fetal monitoring through the use of diagnostic ultrasound. I do so only because it is not generally available to lay readers, nor is it information that is apt to be shared by your doctor. The use of ultrasound for fetal monitoring or any other diagnostic purpose raises some alarming questions that can't be answered by those who employ it. It is another way in which modern obstetrics violates the medical imperative, passed down by Hippocrates, "First, do no harm."

External fetal monitors consist of two bands that are strapped around your abdomen and connected to a monitoring unit that records the device's findings on tape. One band is pressure-sensitive and measures the strength and frequency of your contractions. The other employs ultrasound to determine the condition of the fetus. In most hospitals doctors use fetal monitors routinely, although one study of 70,000 pregnancies found no difference in outcome between monitored and unmonitored patients, and other studies have shown that monitoring results in an increase in infant mortality among the patients monitored. This suggests that, at best, monitoring does no good, and at worst it may do harm.

There is, at this writing, no conclusive evidence directly linking ultrasound to fetal damage, nor is there any hard evidence that it will not cause damage. Unlike X-rays, which impart an electrical charge to matter through a process called *ionization*, ultrasound rays are nonionizing. Proponents of ultrasound seize this as proof that it is not dangerous, but there is no evidence that this defense is valid. In short, I can't prove conclusively that ultrasound may damage your baby, but the doctor who uses it on you can't prove that it won't.

Alice Stewart, a British epidemiologist who heads the Oxford Survey of Childhood Cancers, commented in mid-1983 on "very suspicious hints" that children exposed to ultrasound in the womb may be developing leukemia and other cancers in higher numbers than unexposed children. A World Health Organization report calling for extensive research on the hazards of ultrasound, and restraint in its use, had this to say about benefits versus risks (all italics mine):

Choosing end points for study [of ultrasound] is especially difficult in human subjects. *Latent periods easily could be as long as 20 years in the case of cancer development, or the effect may not be seen for another generation....* Because the human fetus is sensitive to other forms of radiation there is considerable concern that it may also be sensitive to ultrasound.... Animal studies suggest neurologic [sensory, cognitive, and developmental], immunologic, and hematologic possibilities for studies in humans. There is some evidence that if the exposure is within the period of organogenesis, *congenital malformations* may result from exposure to ultrasound in laboratory animals. In general, these end points in animal studies *have been unexplored in humans and should be followed up wherever possible....*

It is not clear at this time whether ultrasound fetal monitoring is beneficial to the mother or fetus in terms of pregnancy outcome and this, above all, should be examined closely; *if there is no generally acknowledged benefit to the monitoring, there is no reason to expose patients to increased costs and possible risk.*

If, despite the concerns that have been raised about leukemia, suppression of the immune response, congenital malformations of the fetus, and other possible effects of ultrasound, your doctor still insists on using it on you, what can you do? I suggest that you tell him you will permit it when he presents you with convincing scientific evidence that it is necessary, that you and your baby will benefit from it, and that it won't harm you or your baby now or 20 years down the road.

He can't very well object to your desire for this reassurance in your own behalf and that of your unborn child. He will also be unable to provide it, because such evidence doesn't exist. Perhaps that will persuade him to do what he should have done in the first place: forget about ultrasound and use his stethoscope instead!

If you have already given birth to a healthy, normal child, you need not be concerned with these prenatal risks until you decide to have another. If you are awaiting the birth of a child, I urge you to study the potential hazards that await you with great care. It is because of risks such as those I have described that I find home birth so appealing. That is why I was overjoyed when both of my own daughters opted to have their babies at home. My own beautiful, healthy grandchildren are now two, three, and five years old, and each of my daughters is due to present me with another. They, too, will be delivered at home.

If you're not ready to accept home birth as an option, and elect to have your child in a hospital, be on your guard. Make good use of what you have learned in this chapter, and in the other books that you read, and you should be able to avoid most of the risks to yourself and your baby that I have described.

Hazards that Lurk in the Hospital Nursery

Although competitive pressures have brought improvements in some hospitals, the probability remains that your baby will be whisked off to the nursery moments after he is born. He will be subjected to a number of procedures, some of them legally mandated in most states, and then compelled to lie there—probably screaming his head off—for at least four hours. Only then, and only once every four hours after that, will you be allowed to breastfeed your baby or give him his bottle, if that is the option you select.

Your obstetrician will waste no time in giving your new baby his first exposure to the chemicals that dominate medical practice in the United States. He'll squirt a few drops of silver nitrate into the baby's eyes. This treatment is predicated on the ridiculous presumption that all mothers must be suspected of having gonorrhea, which may have been transmitted to the baby during delivery. Doctors have, in fact, fostered legislation requiring this treatment in every state.

Doctors reject the argument that the mother could be tested for gonorrhea instead of inflicting silver nitrate on her baby, claiming that this won't do because the test is not 100-percent accurate. That defense is pure nonsense, because the silver nitrate isn't 100-percent effective, either. Whether one is more effective than the other is moot, because if your baby were to develop gonorrheal ophthalmia for either reason, the problem can and will be solved by using antibiotics to treat the disease.

The use of silver nitrate made some sense before antibiotics became available, but the price your baby pays because its use is continued today, when it is no longer needed, is not insignificant. Silver nitrate causes chemical conjunctivitis in 30 to 50 percent of the babies who receive it. Their eyes fill up with thick pus, making it impossible for them to see during the first week or so of life. No one knows what the long-term psychological consequences of this temporary blindness may be. The treatment may also produce blocked tearducts, which necessitates difficult surgical intervention to correct damage done by a senseless procedure. Finally, some doctors—including me—believe that the high incidence of myopia and astigmatism in the United States may be related to the placing of this caustic agent into the delicate, tender membranes of your baby's eyes.

In some states doctors may now substitute antibiotics for the silver nitrate, although there is no evidence that this prophylactic use of antibiotics to prevent gonorrhea is effective. This does eliminate the immediate damage that may be done by silver nitrate, but it also provides the first example of indiscriminate use of antibiotics, which probably will be oft-repeated by your pediatrician and may cause problems for your child later in life.

In many hospitals a second example of indiscriminate use of antibiotics may follow on the heels of the first one. In an effort to prevent the crossinfection that threatens babies in hospital nurseries, many doctors are now giving routine injections of penicillin. Because every use of antibiotics contributes to the possibility of sensitization in later life, it should be avoided unless the treatment is appropriate and essential in dealing with a disease. There is also the risk, in some children, of an allergic shock reaction to antibiotics of all kinds.

When your baby reaches the nursery he will be bathed immediately, and there is a strong probability that the nurse will use hexachlorophene soap. It has been known for many years that hexachlorophene is absorbed through the skin and that it can cause neurologic damage in some children. Yet hospitals continue to use it, despite the risk to your baby, to try to avoid the onus of a bacterial epidemic in their germ-laden nurseries.

What makes this ridiculous, and even reckless, is the fact that hexachlorophene soap and antiseptic preparations afford no advantage over bathing with plain tap water. In five carefully conducted trials involving 150 newborns, 25 infants were bathed with each of four different antiseptics and 50 were bathed with plain water. Bacteriologic samples taken from each group following the initial bath and on the third and fifth days showed that all of the baths were equally effective.

Don't let the hospital expose your baby to a potentially dangerous chemical to reduce the danger of infection when plain water will work just as well!

Another beloved procedure that your infant child will be subjected to is the PKU (phenylketonuria) test. Legally mandated in most states, it is given to determine whether an infant is a victim of a rare form of mental retardation. The condition is caused by an enzyme deficiency, but it occurs in less than one out of 100,000 babies.

The PKU blood test itself is not dangerous, except that it does require insertion of a needle that will open a pathway for the bacteria that abound in every hospital nursery. The problem lies with the test results, which are notoriously inaccurate and result in many false positive findings. If your child is diagnosed as a victim of PKU, he will be placed on a restricted diet composed of protein substitutes that have an offensive taste, tend to cause obesity, and become terribly monotonous. There is disagreement among doctors on how long the diet should be continued. The range is from three years to life. Most doctors who diagnose PKU will not permit the mother to breastfeed.

It is ridiculous, in my judgment, to condemn children to an obnoxious special diet based on a test that may be wrong, for a disease that rarely occurs, when the prescribed diet itself raises serious questions. Seven years ago treatment centers in the United States, Australia, England, and Germany revealed that some children with PKU showed progressive neurologic deterioration "even though their disorder had been diagnosed early and dietary treatment had been promptly instituted." All of these children labeled as having "variant forms of PKU," which differed from the classic form, died.

Unless there is a history of PKU in your family, my advice is to avoid the test and breastfeed your baby, which I believe to be the best treatment anyway, even if he has the disease. If you can't escape the test, and the finding is positive, insist that it be repeated a couple of weeks later to assure that the first result was accurate. If it is still positive, make sure that the doctor determines whether the PKU is the classic or a variant form, and make certain that the diet your child is given is appropriate for its type. Finally, insist on continuing to breastfeed along with the diet, because that's the best overall health protection your child can have.

If the second test is negative, don't fret for years wondering whether the first one might have been right. One of the unfortunate consequences of all forms of indiscriminate mass screening is the emotional trauma parents go through when a false positive reading is given. I have had more than one mother ask me years later, "Do you think 'it' (late talking, late toilet training, etc.) might be PKU?" The same thing happens when a pediatrician tells a parent that a child has "a slight heart murmur."

This sounds threatening, but unless there are other symptoms, they are simply an innocuous finding that does not signify disease.

The list of obscure diseases for which mass screening of newborns is required is steadily expanding, although the requirements vary widely from state to state. Doctors are the prime movers behind this legislation, and in my judgment they are also the prime beneficiaries. It is ridiculous to expose all children and their parents to the physical and emotional risks of screening for diseases that aren't seen more than once in a blue moon.

Also add to the dangers that await your child in the newborn nursery the possible use of bilirubin lights to treat infant jaundice. This is a common condition in newborn babies, and the chances are somewhere between 30 and 50 percent that your baby will be mildly jaundiced. How great that chance is will be determined to a large extent by the degree of obstetric intervention you experience in the delivery process.

It seems that every generation of doctors creates a new set of interventions that create problems that can only be resolved by further intervention. Most of the things a mother goes through when her baby is delivered in a hospital—the analgesia, the anesthesia, the induction of labor, all of the drugs—increase the chance that her infant will develop jaundice, because it is one of their side effects.

Many doctors routinely give vitamin K to newborn babies because they have been taught that infants are born with a deficiency of this vitamin, which influences how rapidly the baby's blood will clot. That's nonsense, unless the mother is severely malnourished; but most doctors do it anyway. Administration of vitamin K to the newborn may produce jaundice, which prompts the pediatrician to treat it with bilirubin lights (phototherapy). These lights expose the baby to a dozen documented hazards that may require still further treatment and possibly affect him for the rest of his life.

Bilirubin is the bile pigment found in the bloodstream,

which your doctor will probably describe as a potential source of brain damage through transfer of the pigment from the bloodstream to the central nervous system. Actually, bilirubin is a normal breakdown pattern of the red blood cells. This breakdown converts them into bilirubin, which is what gives your infant the jaundiced, yellow coloring. The condition is not threatening except in rare instances when it is very high or rapidly rising on the first day of life. This is usually caused by Rh sensitization and requires treatment with bilirubin lights or exchange transfusions. The transfusion simply replaces your infant's blood with other blood that is not contaminated with bilirubin, while the bilirubin lights hasten its excretion. Light in the blue part of the spectrum, which can be supplied artificially in the hospital nursery, or naturally by the ultraviolet rays in sunlight, oxidizes bilirubin more rapidly so that it can be excreted through the liver.

If jaundice does not appear until after the first day of life, the risks of treating it outweigh the benefits. The bilirubin is normally excreted naturally, and the process of excretion can be hastened by exposing your child to natural sunlight, but it may take a week or two to get rid of all of it.

Despite the normal and nonthreatening nature of most cases of infant jaundice, doctors usually insist on treating the condition with bilirubin lights, rather than permitting natural sunlight to do the job. Now your child's health *is* threatened by using phototherapy to treat a nonthreatening condition! Responsible medical authorities have reported that phototherapy for infant jaundice may be responsible for increased mortality, particularly in very small infants. The higher risk of death results from lung problems (respirator distress syndrome) and hemorrhage. Infant deaths have also been reported from aspiration of pads placed over their eyes to protect them from the lights.

Although your doctor will probably assure you that treatment with bilirubin lights is completely safe, no one actually knows what the long-term effects may be, and plenty of short-term effects have already been identified. They include irritability and sluggishness, diarrhea, lactase deficiency, intestinal irritation, dehydration, feeding problems, riboflavin deficiency, disturbance of the bilirubin-albumin relationship, poor visual orientation with possible diminished responsiveness to parents, and DNA-modifying effects.

If, because of a misguided cesarean, excessive weight control during pregnancy, or for other reasons, you have a low-birth-weight baby, you will have to contend with the treatment he gets in the neonatal intensive care nursery. Doctors and hospitals take intense pride in these facilities and all of the technological wizardry they employ—an attitude that mystifies me, because there is no evidence that they benefit the children who are isolated in them.

They do, however, expose your child to additional risks. If your low-birth-weight child is sent to intensive care, he will be separated from you immediately after birth and placed in a radiant warmer. This involves some element of risk, because babies have been burned in them. The risk that should cause the greatest concern, however, arises when your child is given oxygen while he is in this incubator.

Failure of your doctor to limit the flow rate of oxygen properly can in premature babies result in a disease known as *retrolental fibroplasia*, the leading cause of blindness in children. To avoid this, the oxygen level in your baby's blood must be closely monitored, which means drawing blood, and that in turn can produce a condition known as *iatrogenic anemia*. One intervention continues to lead to another, and the baby may need a blood transfusion, which exposes him to the risk of acquiring serum hepatitis or AIDS.

If your child is placed on oxygen in intensive care, let your doctor know that you are aware of these risks and that they are causing you great concern. That may forestall any carelessness on the part of the medical personnel.

CIRCUMCISION AND OTHER SURGERY—UNNECESSARY PROCEDURES

The odds are high that if you have a male baby your doctor will recommend that he be circumcised. About 1,500,000 circumcisions are performed each year. That represents about 80 percent of all the male babies that are born in the United States. If performed for other than religious reasons, it is a useless, unnecessary, and potentially dangerous procedure.

Every generation of doctors has found a new excuse for circumcision, despite the fact that even the American Academy of Pediatrics has advised that "There is no absolute medical indication for circumcision of the newborn." If your doctor suggests circumcision for your baby boy, ask him why he wants to expose the poor kid to the pain, the possibility of infection or hemorrhage, and the risk of death from surgery that has no medical justification.

Although it is not likely that they will be performed immediately after birth, you should also beware of two other surgical procedures for conditions that may exist at birth. The first of these is the umbilical hernia, a small defect in the abdominal muscle that permits the abdominal contents to protrude. The condition is quite common and can usually be expected to correct itself before your baby's first birthday. However, even if it doesn't, surgery should not be considered until your child is three to five years old, because there is still a good chance that the condition will correct itself.

Finally, there is the possibility that your baby may be

born with an undescended testicle, and your doctor will recommend surgery to bring it down. The need to do so is dubious, at best. Some doctors maintain that it is essential because of the threat that cancer may develop in the undescended testicle. That reasoning may seem persuasive, but it shouldn't be, because the mortality rate from the surgery is higher than the potential mortality rate from testicular cancer. Consequently, it is safer for your child to leave the undescended testicle alone. It is another matter if your child has two undescended testicles. In that event surgery deserves serious consideration because sterility is almost inevitable if neither of your child's testes is in its proper place.

I have tried to forewarn you in this chapter of all of the risks that you and your child will face if you are hospitalized when he is born. Yet these are only the immediate dangers. In addition, there are psychological and nutritional risks that arise from your separation from your child and the interference of hospital procedures with normal breastfeeding. I will cover these in subsequent chapters.

5

Proper Nutrition for Health and Growth

Your most important contribution to the future health of your child will be the attention you give to your own diet during pregnancy and to proper nutrition for your baby after he is born. Because your pediatrician has little knowledge and even less interest in nutrition, you will have to become your own expert where your child's diet is concerned.

Your first and most important nutritional decision—whether you will breastfeed your baby or not—will affect his health and development in infancy and for the rest of his life. Unfortunately, most obstetricians and pediatricians fail to emphasize the importance of breastfeeding strongly enough and to inform you fully, if at all, of the comparative shortcomings of bottlefeeding formula milk. It is essential, therefore, that you inform yourself.

Breastfeeding lays the foundation for healthy physical and emotional growth and provides your child and yourself with many additional benefits as well. Here are some of the benefits of breastfeeding that are stimulating a promising resurgence of this womanly art in the United States.

1. Mother's milk, time-tested for millions of years, is the best nutrient for babies because it is nature's perfect food. It provides your child with all of the nutrients he needs for healthy growth for at least the first six months of life, and all responsible nutritional and pediatric authorities acknowledge its superiority over both infant formulas and cow's milk.

Cow's milk is deficient in iron and should not be given to babies for at least six months. Even then it should be introduced with caution, because many babies—perhaps as many as 15 percent—are allergic to cow's milk. It should be suspected as the potential cause of many illnesses.

Bottlefeeding with infant formula is also less than satisfactory from a nutritional standpoint, even though the manufacturers fortify their products with vitamins and minerals and maintain that their products are as nutritious as mother's milk. If you breastfeed your baby there is no danger that some essential nutrient will be omitted from your milk, but that can't be said for manufactured infant formula. The manufacturers not only *can* fail but *have* failed to include essential ingredients, with disastrous consequences for the infants who were fed their products. Classic examples were the lack of vitamin B_6 in SMA formula, which led to a pyroxidine deficiency and convulsions in the infants who received it, and the production of Neo-Mull-Soy with an inadequate salt content, which resulted in failure to thrive.

Bottlefeeding with infant formulas also predisposes infants to lifelong obesity because the products provide the wrong kind of nutrients. Human milk is 1.3 percent protein; cow's milk and infant formulas are 3.3 percent protein or more. That's why one study of 250 full-term infants at six weeks of age found that 60 percent of the bottlefed babies were overweight, compared to 19 percent of those who were breastfed. Excess protein places an unduly heavy load on the kidneys, and some children gain weight faster because they retain more fluid.

Finally, breastfed babies are permitted to eat until they are satisfied, and you have no ability or need to measure the quantity of milk that your child takes. Formula-fed babies are usually placed on a fixed schedule, with a measured amount of milk given at each feeding. Too often, mothers feel a responsibility to encourage their baby to take the full scheduled feeding, making him drink six or eight ounces when he was satisfied with four. I'll have more to say about the relationship between infant overfeeding and obesity later on.

2. A breastfed baby gains from his mother's milk a natural immunity to many allergies and infections that is denied to babies who are bottlefed. Mother's milk contains unique substances that inhibit the growth of bacteria and viruses, affording your baby critical protection against disease during the most hazardous months of his life.

3. The bonding of mother and child is regarded as essential to your baby's emotional development, and it provides emotional rewards for you, as well. The nurturing that breastfeeding supplies is the ideal way to establish this bond almost from the moment of birth. Unless you have received excessive drugs during delivery, which also affected your baby, his desire to begin nursing should be at its peak within 20-30 minutes after birth. From that moment on he should be nursed when he gives evidence of the desire to do so. At the outset this may be as many as 20 times a day.

The emotional and psychological rewards of breastfeeding cannot be overstressed. You and your baby will sacrifice one of the most beneficial of human experiences if you fail to breastfeed. Dr. Grantly Dick-Read, regarded by many as the father of today's natural birth movement, said it well: "The newborn baby has only three demands. They are warmth in the arms of its mother, food from her breasts, and security in the knowledge of her presence. Breastfeeding satisfies all three."

Newborn babies should be fed when they are hungry, not on some arbitrary schedule. That's one of the additional shortcomings of postnatal procedure in most hospitals, which I alluded to earlier. Too often, mothers and babies are required to conform to a four-hour feeding schedule, simply because that is more convenient for the hospital staff. This is not good for your baby and it is not good for you. Your baby's hunger is regulated by his need for food, not by the nursery clock. He should be fed when he wants to be fed, whether that's once every hour or once every four.

If your baby is born in a hospital, try to secure permission to keep him in your room so that you can feed him as often as he desires and give him the nurturing that will help bonding take place. If this is not permitted, demand that he be brought to you when he is hungry, not every four hours. Also caution your doctor to insist that no supplementary feeding be given your baby in the nursery. Some nurses can't resist the temptation to shove a bottle of formula into a baby's mouth when he cries, even when the baby is being breastfed. This may quell his appetite when you are feeding him, and you don't want him to have the formula, so it is appropriate to insist that when your baby cries the nurses bring him to you instead.

4. *Not to be overlooked in deciding whether you will breastfeed your baby are several factors of specific importance to you.* If you begin nursing your baby within a few minutes after delivery, it will help prevent hemorrhage because his sucking will cause your uterus to contract, hastening its return to its normal condition which reduces the flow of blood.

Mothers who breastfeed are able to return to their normal weight with greater ease than those who abandon this phase of the reproductive cycle by resorting to bottlefeeding. Typically, about nine pounds of a mother's weight gain during pregnancy is body fat, which is believed to accumulate to enable you to produce milk for the baby after his birth. If you breastfeed, this excess fat will be consumed in the process. If you don't, heroic measures may be required to restore your normal weight.

5. If your baby is totally breastfed, it will provide you with contraceptive protection, in most cases, for at least six months, and in some instances for as long as 2½ years. The act of breastfeeding causes your reproductive cycle to move into a dormant stage, and you are unlikely to have menstrual periods for seven months or more after the delivery of your baby or to become pregnant until after your periods resume. Sheila Kippley, author of an excellent book on breastfeeding, examined data on American women whose babies were totally breastfed and found an average of 14.6 months without menstrual periods after their babies were born.

While this means of contraception is not completely reliable, it is probably as effective as any of the others, and no risks are involved. Remember, though, that occasional, haphazard breastfeeding won't do the trick. If you breastfeed your baby only occasionally, and give him a bottle of formula at other times, you probably won't receive the contraceptive benefit that exclusive breastfeeding will provide.

I get a lot of questions from new mothers about how often their babies should be fed, how long they should be fed, and how much they should eat. My answer—whether your baby is breastfed or bottlefed—is that the baby is boss. Feed him when he seems irritable, let him nurse until he loses interest, and don't be concerned about whether he is eating too little or too much.

If you breastfeed, your baby will consume 80-90 percent of the available milk in about four minutes of feeding on each breast. However, a longer period of nursing is advisable for emotional reasons and to stimulate the production of milk. The act of nursing, even when it is only minimally productive in providing additional food, stimulates lactation and increases the production of milk. If you limit the period of nursing unduly, or fail to nurse your baby often enough, lactation may decrease to the point at which you are not producing as much milk as your baby requires.

The emotional reasons for extending the nursing periods are very important. My friends in the LaLeche League, to which I was medical advisor for many years, tell me that more mothers would breastfeed if they were aware of the wondrous relationship it establishes between mother and child. Some mothers, they say, are also intimidated by the misconception that breastfeeding is inevitably a difficult, uncomfortable, unmanageable nuisance. There is no doubt that many mothers have that concern, but in my experience, once they experience the pleasures of breastfeeding, it is quickly dispelled. If you are undecided about whether to breastfeed your baby, I urge you to read *The Womanly Art of Breastfeeding*, published by the LaLeche League International, Inc., 9616 Minneapolis Ave., Franklin Park, IL 60131, and *Breast-feeding and Natural Child Spacing; The Ecology of Natural Mothering*, by Sheila Kippley, Harper and Row, 1974; Penguin, 1975.

It is not necessary to give supplementary water to a breastfed baby, nor are supplemental vitamins required. Babies who are fed infant formula don't need supplementary vitamins, either, because these products are fortified with them. A healthy child does not benefit from excess vitamins and may be damaged by them.

DON'T START SOLID FOODS TOO EARLY

Breastfed babies do not require solid foods during the first year of life and should not be given any during at least the first six months of life. Bottlefed babies should not be given solid foods for at least four months. Until the infant is four months old, much of the solid food he eats passes through his body undigested. The intestines are not yet well enough developed to process solid food, particularly protein. For example, the enzyme that is needed to process rice cereal is not present, in quantities adequate to digest it, until your baby is four months old. Solid foods should also be avoided in the first months of life because the baby's allergy defenses are not yet fully developed, and there is also a higher incidence of choking because the art of swallowing is still being mastered.

Solid foods should be introduced gradually into the infant's diet: fruit or cereal is usually given first, then meat. Avoid commercially prepared baby foods to the extent that you can, not only because they are more expensive, but because they are less nutritious after being processed to death.

Your baby will fare best if you prepare his food yourself. Use fresh fruits, vegetables, and meats, because canned and frozen foods contain varying levels of salt and other additives such as nitrites and monosodium glutamate. Wash the food carefully and make sure it is thoroughly cooked. Then grind it, puree it, mash it, or put it in a blender, and spoon it in.

Many mothers have found that babies respond well to mashed fresh bananas or cooked yams as their first food. Babies seem to like the flavor, and they are easy to prepare. Cereals can be introduced by giving your baby bits of natural, whole-grain bread. This will do as well as cooked cereal, although a lot of the bread will probably land on the floor until your baby learns how to manage it. If you feed him cooked cereal, be sure it is the natural, whole-grain variety, not the processed variety from which nutritious ingredients have been removed and potentially harmful chemicals added.

Eggs, because they often cause allergic reactions, should be avoided until your baby is at least a year old. Introduce hard-boiled eggs first, feeding only the mashed-up yolk. If there is no negative reaction after a couple of weeks, it is time to try feeding eggs scrambled without milk. Cow's milk should also be avoided until your baby is at least a year old and then introduced gradually. Observe your baby closely to be sure that there is no allergic physical or behavioral reaction, such as excessive crying or fussiness.

A hidden benefit of preparing your own baby food may be the influence it will have on the diet consumed by the others in the family. They will share in your efforts to provide your baby with a nutritious, natural, well-balanced diet. However, unless you want them to eat elsewhere, don't expect them to enjoy their dinner if it, too, is pureed.

Don't allow your pediatrician or anyone else to try to persuade you to use commercial baby foods for reasons of safety. The baby food manufacturers are not above attempting to frighten mothers who feed their children table food rather than their canned products. A pamphlet that did this, *Dear Mother*, put out by the manufacturers of Beech Nut baby foods, compelled even the staid American Academy of Pediatrics committee on nutrition to protest. The committee said it deplored industry "scare" tactics and was concerned that some material from scientific publications had been taken out of context.

"We are not in agreement with implied excessive dangers in home preparation of foods," the committee declared. "Obviously care should be taken in the preparation and storage of infant foods, but the likelihood of home-prepared fresh foods being toxic is remote."

CHILDREN'S APPETITES VARY

Parents sometimes become overly preoccupied with how much their child is eating. If the pediatrician has said that a bottlefed baby should be getting six ounces of formula at each feeding, mother will struggle to get him to consume the last half-ounce. As the child gets older, there may be repeated battles at the dinner table to get him to join the clean-plate club. This is a mistake, and the worries are unnecessary, because no child—unless he or she is suffering from anorexia nervosa—will ever starve to death if food is available.

The size of a child's appetite will vary from day to day and year to year for a variety of reasons. It can be affected by his level of activity, by his fondness for the food he is served, and by the intake he requires if he is in the midst of a spurt in growth. The child, whether he is a baby or in his teens, will eat what he needs.

Children are often condemned to adult obesity because they were overfed as children. Studies of infants at various ages up to 18 months show more than 70 percent getting excess calories, some as much as 250 percent of the recommended daily allowance for normal nutritional and energy needs. It is also estimated that 30 percent of all school age children are overweight.

This becomes troublesome in later life because adult obesity results from excessive production of fat cells in the early childhood years. The number of fat cells increases from birth to two years and again at puberty. An overfed child may have 75 trillion fat cells when he becomes an adult, compared with 27 trillion for a child who was fed an adequate but not excessive diet. This difference is important because weight gain in adults is not due to an increase in the number of fat cells but to an increase in their size. If too many fat cells have been produced in childhood, they remain in the body for life, waiting to be filled up when the adult eats a high-calorie meal or a chocolate eclair.

One basic rule should be your guide in your effort to provide sound nutrition for your children and others in your family: *the more any food is processed, the less nutritious it becomes*. Virtually all foods are most nutritious when they are served in their raw, natural state. If they must be cooked, the duration of cooking should be as short as possible. That's one reason why the Chinese stir-frying method is so attractive. Fresh fruits and vegetables are more nutritious than the same varieties after they have been cooked and canned.

At the opposite end of the spectrum are the "convenience" foods that have become so popular in the United States, and breads and cereals made from refined flour and loaded with refined sugar. The "empty calories" they provide, and the chemical additives used to color, flavor, stabilize, and preserve them, are the last thing your child needs. Keep that in mind as you plan the meals you prepare for your family. Serve fresh, natural foods prepared from scratch and avoid processed commercial products such as packaged "TV dinners."

If you stick with natural foods and cook them as little as possible, little is required to assure your family of a healthy diet other than the application of common sense. Don't concern yourself with all of the unproven medical theories about the hazards of feeding your child eggs, or dairy products, or any other natural, unprocessed food. Provide a varied, balanced diet and your family will get all of the nutrients it needs. The basic guideline for a daily diet that most nutritionists would suggest for pre-adolescents is this: three servings of milk or milk products, or an alternative source of protein; two servings of meat, cheese, eggs, peanut butter, beans, or other protein source; four or more servings of fresh fruits and vegetables; and four or more servings of breads made from unrefined flour and cereal grains. However, it is worth noting that a child's entire nutritional need, including protein and calcium, can be met without milk or milk products.

Remember that breakfast is the most important meal of the day. If your child skips it, he will be more susceptible to infection and also to fatigue, which may affect his general health and hamper his work in school. Be sure that he eats wholesome food for breakfast, not sugar-laden junk. Don't let him form the habit of putting sugar on his cereal, and don't introduce him to the sugar-coated cereals that the breakfast food manufacturers push so vigorously on TV.

Remember, too, that it is tradition, not nutrition, that is responsible for the American habit of breakfasting on cereal, pancakes, bacon, and eggs. Your child's nutritional needs will be as well served—perhaps better served—if you give him wholesome leftovers from the dinner you had the night before. I've often thought it ironic that many Americans are appalled by the fact that Mexican children breakfast on a bowl of beans and the Chinese on a bowl of brown rice. Both are healthy foods that contain a wealth of protein and vitamins. Meanwhile, the typical American kid is eating an expensive commercial cereal that has been processed to death and loaded with refined sugar, yielding empty calories that do him little good.

KIDS DON'T HAVE TO EAT EVERYTHING

Don't be upset if your child takes an instant dislike to some foods—particularly vegetables. As long as he is getting a basic diet, with all of the food groups represented, it isn't imperative that he eat every vegetable in your produce merchant's bins. The classic source of mealtime friction seems to be spinach, which most kids hate and most parents apparently believe to be an essential source of iron and calcium. Actually, while spinach is rich in these minerals, they are present in a form that is difficult to digest, and spinach is a poor energy source. So, don't push spinach if your child doesn't like it. If he has an aversion to *all* vegetables, try concealing them in stews, soups, or breads, and encourage him to try eating them raw.

Don't get so locked into conventional mealtimes that you can't be flexible if your child seems hungriest at some other hour. His bodily clock may not be regulated by Emily Post. If his appetite suddenly slacks off, bear in mind that it may simply be a natural reduction in his food requirements, but consider also the possibility that he is eating too many snacks. If it proves to be the snacks, make certain that those which are available to him are healthful ones such as fresh fruit, raisins, nuts, seeds, yogurt, raw vegetables, and milk.

I'll conclude this chapter with a warning about the potential nutritional consequences if it becomes necessary for your child to be hospitalized. It is here, on their own turf, that the nutritional indifference of doctors is most clearly demonstrated. That's why it is important for you to observe closely how well he eats during his hospital stay and what kind of diet he receives.

Studies have found that up to half of the patients confined to hospitals suffer from malnutrition within a few days. That's not because hospital food is necessarily bad; much of it, in fact, is pretty good. It is because doctors are so enamored with medical technology—lab tests and X-rays—that require their patients to fast or eat severely restricted diets. Some patients literally waste away from malnutrition while their doctors subject them to an elaborate series of tests in an effort to determine what is wrong with them. By the time the doctor is through with his tests, malnutrition may have become the patient's most serious problem.

One study of children's nutrition in a New York hospital found that two-thirds of 200 children had a nutrition problem. Those who conducted the study said that this did not surprise them but that they "were somewhat chagrined to find out what many physicians don't know concerning the details of pediatric nutrition." A majority of the primary physicians caring for the children had never had a nutrition course of any kind!

I don't know why they should have been surprised. Several years ago the chairman of the American Medical Association committee on nutrition noted "... the growing suspicion that a great many people in the nation's hospitals are unwillingly becoming the victims of physician-induced malnutrition and outright starvation.... It is not due to wilful neglect on the physician's part; rather it is due to his lack of understanding of the whole new science of nutrition."

This criticism did not pass unnoticed within the AMA. It solved the problem to its own satisfaction, if not to mine or yours, by abandoning the committee on nutrition!

There is no more important action that you can take to raise a healthy child, or one in which you can place less reliance on the medical profession, than making sure that he eats the right kinds of food in the appropriate quantities, and avoids those that will do him harm.

6

What You Should Expect of Your Child

Most baby books dwell at length on the developmental landmarks of early childhood—sitting, standing, crawling, walking—and the host of behavioral concerns that will surface as your child grows older. These milestones are of legitimate interest to proud parents, but only rarely should they be a matter of concern, and I don't need a whole book to give you my advice about them. I'll do it in one sentence: unless there is something obviously wrong with your child, don't worry about how soon he sits, stands, crawls, or walks.

If this is your first child, you will be strongly tempted to compare his progress with that of other children his age. I know that nothing I write will keep you from doing that, but I hope I can convince you that such comparisons are more apt to mislead than to inform. During the first few years of life the development of individual children varies so widely that comparisons are meaningless. However, if you want a rule of thumb, try this: most children sit with support at 6–8 months, sit without support at 8–10 months, walk at 12–18 months, talk at 18–24 months, ride a tricycle at 3 years, and copy a square at 4 years. Having said that, let me urge you to resist the temptation to boast if your child reaches any of these milestones at an earlier age or to worry if his development is delayed. At some point in their development all normal children arrive at the same place, and whether it is early or late makes no difference.

Sooner or later your children will learn to do what you expect of them if your expectations are realistic. All of us know, but we sometimes forget, that all children do not learn at the same rate, within the same time frame, with the same ease; nor can they be expected to reach a uniform level of achievement by the time they become adults. That knowledge, unfortunately, does not prevent us from having grand expectations of our own children, which begin while they are still in the crib. Nor does it keep us from making behavioral comparisons with other children that are both meaningless and dangerous. Today's "early bloomer" may be the backward child of tomorrow, and vice versa.

Our rosy expectations of our kids are beneficial if they encourage us to give them the attention and support they need to achieve the potential they have. They can also be devastating to our child's development and self-image if our expectations exceed his potential, or if we lack the patience to allow his skills and interests to develop naturally during the formative years.

It is sometimes difficult for parents with high expectations, who may themselves be high achievers, to remember that the occupation of children is to play and to learn. We must learn to accept the fact that during their developmental years children cannot be expected to exhibit adult behavior. More likely, many of the things they do will seem almost calculated to drive you up the wall. Nothing I have to say in this chapter will make your child's annoying behavior any less worrisome or exasperating, but it may be easier to live with if you understand what's normal and where the child is coming from.

PHYSICAL BEHAVIOR THAT CONCERNS PARENTS

First let's separate physical behavior from emotional behavior. What are the physical things that parents most commonly worry about? All babies, often to the initial distress of their parents, cough, grunt, belch, hiccup, sneeze, pass gas, spit up, and vomit. You may worry about this at first and wonder whether it indicates some deficiency in your child's diet. You needn't, because as long as the baby is eating right and not losing weight you can regard all of this behavior as normal.

While we're on the subject of infantile sounds, let me caution you also not to get hung up on burping. Somewhere in the distant past some mother found that her baby was less apt to spit up his lunch if she patted him on the back until excess air was released from his stomach. This procedure has become such a ritual that some new mothers appear to believe that their child will not survive if he doesn't burp loudly after every meal. In fact, there's nothing carved in stone that says your baby has to burp. Some babies swallow a lot of air and readily produce an earsplitting burp. Others swallow very little and don't need to burp at all. If you find that burping after a meal keeps your baby from spitting up, you may want to encourage him a bit, but don't make a production of it. There is no medical reason why he has to burp at all.

While we're on the subject, let me say a word about colic. This is the name mothers and doctors give to a phenomenon that usually occurs before three months of age. A previously placid and contented baby suddenly begins drawing up his legs and having paroxysms of screaming. It may surprise you, considering the eon that babies have been on earth, but there isn't a shred of scientific evidence indicating what causes it. However, the word *colic* is a convenient term for doctors, who use it to explain crying that they can't explain.

Some medical textbooks refer to "gas" in the intestines, caused by excessive fermentation of carbohydrates, as a possible cause. But then they note that removing the carbohydrates doesn't relieve the condition, which seems to cast grave doubts on this explanation. The simple truth is that many mothers and most doctors talk about "colic" as uncontrollable crying caused by "gas" in the baby's stomach. Scientists say that they don't know what causes it. I'm with the scientists. I don't know, either!

Crying is the second worrisome behavior that appears at birth. The first cry you hear is reassuring, but from then on crying is something every parent could cheerfully do without. Over the years doctors have given parents a lot of bad advice about what to do when their baby cries, and a lot of kids have suffered because of it.

I was amused recently to come across a book published in 1894 by Dr. Luther Emmett Holt, who is generally regarded as the father of pediatrics. The book, *Care and Feeding of Children*, went through more than 75 printings and was published in three languages, and upon reading it, I was reminded of where pediatricians got a lot of their bad advice. Here, in his question-answer style, is what he had to say about crying:

When is crying useful?
> In the newly born infant the cry expands the lungs, and it is necessary that it should be repeated for a few minutes every day to keep them well expanded.

How much crying is normal for a very young baby?
> From 15 to 30 minutes a day.

What is the nature of this cry?
> It is loud and strong. Infants get red in the face with it; in fact, it is a scream. This is necessary for health. It is the baby's exercise.

What is the cry of indulgence or from habit?
> This is often heard even in very young infants, who cry to be rocked, to be carried about, sometimes for a light in the room, for a bottle to suck, or for the continuance of any other bad habit which has been acquired.

How can we be sure that a child is crying to be indulged?
> If it stops immediately when it gets what it wants, and cries when it is withdrawn or withheld.

How is an infant to be managed that cries from temper or to be indulged?
> It should simply be allowed to cry it out. A second struggle is rarely necessary.

At what age may playing with babies be begun?
> Never until four months, and better not until six months. The less of it at any time, the better for the infant.

What harm is done by playing with very young babies?
> They are made nervous and irritable, sleep badly, and suffer in other respects.

Dr. Holt also recommended feeding at regular intervals, putting children to bed at exactly the same time every day and evening, stopping night feedings at five months, and not rocking a baby because it is "useless and sometimes injurious." He also maintained that under no circumstances should a child be allowed to sleep in its mother's bed.

CHILDREN CRY BECAUSE THEY HAVE PROBLEMS

Much of Dr. Holt's advice is still accepted by many pediatricians. Study it, and then do the opposite. Children cry because they are hungry, or lonely, or tired, or wet, or in pain. Compassionate people do not withhold comfort from adults who are crying, for whatever reason. Why in heaven's name should a loving parent withhold comfort from a little child? If your child cries, don't let it continue. Pick him up and find out why. If he cries at night because he is lonely or afraid, take him into your bed.

Psychologists and psychiatrists always give me a bad time when I make that last recommendation. I recall being on the Phil Donahue show with Tine Thevenin, author of *The Family Bed*, and a psychiatrist who was invoking the Oedipus complex and other pet theories to try to put her down. Donahue turned to me for my opinion, and I told him I agreed with the psychiatrist. I said that psychiatrists should not take their children to bed with them, but that it was quite all right for everyone else!

Bowel habits, diarrhea, constipation, and toilet training are also parental concerns that begin at birth and continue through the years. Many first-time mothers are inordinately concerned with the appearance and condition of their baby's stools, particularly if the baby is being breastfed. The color and consistency of a baby's stools vary considerably depending on his diet. Breastfed babies, for example, usually have stools that resemble loose scrambled eggs. This is not diarrhea; it is perfectly normal and not a matter of concern. There is a danger, though, that your pediatrician may use this normal condition as an excuse to switch your child from breastfeeding to formula milk.

If that happens, pay no attention to him. The most sensible rule to follow is this: if your child is thriving and gaining weight, don't worry about the consistency of his stools, whether they are extremely loose or as hard as marbles. You need to be concerned only if he is not thriving, is losing weight, or if the stools are bloody. In that case, see a doctor. However, if this does become necessary, be wary of medications unless your doctor is able to diagnose a specific cause. Pediatricians are inveterate stool-gazers, inclined to treat loose stools with opiates such as Lomotil. In the absence of a specific disease, a more sensible course, which really doesn't require medical supervision, is to look for food allergies and then eliminate the offending foods. The most likely food is cow's milk.

This is also true of constipation. There is no magic number of bowel movements your child should have and no reason to be concerned if he fails to have at least one every day. If your child seems to be constipated, look for the cause in his diet and see a doctor only if the constipation is accompanied by pain or bleeding.

As for toilet training, pay no attention to medical advice, because your pediatrician doesn't know any more about it than you do. It's a family affair. It doesn't make any difference, except in terms of your own convenience, whether you train your child early, late, or neither of the above. Some children train readily. Others don't, and I have no magic formula you can use if you have one of those. My daughters have, though. They turned to their mother for advice on training their children!

The emotional behaviors of children that may provoke frustration and anger in parents are almost endless, from the "terrible twos" to the "turbulent teens." What you must remember, when your nerves get frayed, is that they all stem from developmental processes without which your child could never become a functioning adult. Moreover, physical punishment is rarely, if ever, the solution.

Your immediate reaction is likely to be anger when your toddling child jerks the cloth from a table and smashes your most cherished vase. If it is, you must learn to control it, because at that age hasty physical punishment won't solve the problem; it will merely confuse your child. A more appropriate response will be to remind yourself that the child isn't being deliberately naughty. He's simply exercising the normal curiosity that will enable him to learn and trying out his newfound motor skills. Then, begin firmly but not angrily to teach him the word *no*, and put the rest of your cherished objects out of reach.

PUNISHMENT IS NOT THE SOLUTION

Virtually all disturbing childhood behaviors stem from some emotional cause. Your response is not to punish the child but to isolate the cause. Often, the child you have finally toilet-trained after a long struggle will suddenly begin to wet his pants again. This isn't deliberate, because no child really enjoys wet pants or the negative maternal response they evoke. It is virtually certain, when this happens, that the child is responding to some environmental stress. Don't spank your child; try to identify and eliminate the stress.

Remember, if your child suddenly becomes violent with his playmates, or becomes a discipline problem in school, that he is probably reacting to some situation or problem that is beyond his control. It could be illness, exhaustion, hunger, visual or hearing defects, or simply a reaction to turmoil at home. It may even be a response to his deteriorating self-image because you have unrealistic expectations of him. If so, he won't respond positively to punishment. Emotional support and constant displays of love and affection are more apt to be the cure.

Children must, of course, be guided toward responsible adult behavior, but parents shouldn't expect them to achieve it all at once. Nor is there any convincing evidence that it can be effectively achieved by employing the old maxim "spare the rod and spoil the child." Corporal punishment at any age confuses and traumatizes the child, because he can't understand why the mother and father he loves, and who are supposed to love him, are suddenly raging at him and causing physical pain. He is made to feel insecure, resentful, and even worthless, and the consequence may be psychological harm.

The impact of physical punishment on child development has been studied extensively, and the consensus of this research is that violence damages both parent and child. It fails to teach children *what to do* and yields only a temporary benefit, if that, in teaching them *what not to do*. I won't deny that I've raised my hand in anger on occasion, but for the most part I have tried to achieve the desired end with my own children through the use of example and the provision of tender, loving encouragement. I am more than satisfied with the results, I hope and trust that my grandchildren, likewise, will rarely endure physical punishment of any kind.

SOME MAXIMS ABOUT CHILDHOOD BEHAVIOR

If you become so frustrated with any aspect of your child's behavior that you are tempted to discipline him physically, restrain yourself. Consider alternative means of behavior modification that may be more effective. There are many alternatives to violence, but the subject is too vast to be dealt with here. Your local bookstore is certain to have a shelf full of sound advice, so all I'll provide here is a handful of maxims about child behavior that I have developed for my patients over the years.

- Children aren't adults, so don't expect them to behave as though they were.

- Children learn by doing, so don't expect to approve of everything they do.

- It is a rare child whose behavior equals his parents' expectations.

- Children are more likely to do as you do than to do as you say.

- Adolescence is a time when children learn to be adults by trying their wings. They may need a leash, but never a cage.

- It is often less important for parents to control their children's behavior than it is for them to control their own.

- Children *react* to anger; they *respond* to love and affection.

- The pain you inflict on your children will probably be inflicted on theirs.

A secure and loving home environment and emotional stability within the family appear to be the major elements in overcoming some of the specific behaviors that concern or displease parents. These include thumb sucking, nail biting, nose picking, rocking and head banging, bed wetting, and erratic sleep habits. There are a host of folk treatments for these common annoyances, some of which seem to work for some children, but there is no specific medical "cure" for any of them.

You can deal most successfully with these problems if you refrain from making an issue of them, pay close attention to the emotional needs of your child, make sure that he knows you love him, whatever he does, and exert yourself to make him feel secure. If you develop that kind of warm relationship with him, you'll do more than eliminate annoying habits. You'll be rewarded with a happy, confident, emotionally stable child!

7

Fever: *Your Body's Defense against Disease*

Do you worry when your child has a fever and reach for the telephone to let your doctor know right away? Many parents do, because medical professionals—doctors *and* nurses—have led them to believe that all fevers are dangerous. Doctors have also reinforced the mistaken notion that the height of a child's temperature is a measure of how sick he is. That's why fever is the symptom that produces about 30 percent of the patients a pediatrician sees.

When you telephone your pediatrician to tell him your child is sick his first question, almost invariably, is "Have you taken his temperature?" Whether you tell him 101 or 104, he'll probably tell you to give the kid an aspirin and bring him to the office. This ritual is almost universal among pediatricians. I suspect that some of them perform it by rote and would offer the same advice if you told him your child's temperature was 110! What troubles me is that they ask the wrong question and give the wrong advice. The very fact that fever is their first concern implies that there is something implicitly dangerous about fever itself. Then, when they prescribe aspirin, you are led to the inevitable conclusion that it is necessary and desirable to treat your child with drugs to bring the fever down.

This charade continues when you take your child to

the doctor's office. In most practices the first thing the nurse does is to take his temperature and write it on his chart. There's nothing wrong with that. An elevated temperature does offer a diagnostic clue that can be important in the context of everything else the doctor learns during his subsequent examination. The problem is that the presence of fever is too often given more importance than that. When the doctor finally arrives in the examining room he is apt to look at the chart, assume an expression of benign concern, and say gravely, "Hmmm, 102 degrees. Well, now, we'd better do something about that!"

That's nonsense—misleading nonsense—because the presence of fever, by itself, does not mean that he must or should do anything at all. Unless there are additional symptoms such as extreme listlessness, abnormal behavior, respiratory difficulty, and others that could indicate the presence of serious diseases such as diphtheria and meningitis, your doctor should tell you there is nothing to worry about and send you and your child home.

It is not surprising, in view of this misleading preoccupation of doctors with fever, that the vast majority of parents questioned in surveys fear it greatly and that their degree of concern increases with each degree of temperature registered on the thermometer. Rarely is this concern justified. You'll be spared a lot of parental anguish, and your child will avoid needless and potentially harmful tests, X-rays, and medication, if you keep in mind some basic facts about fever. These are truths that every doctor should know, that many seem to ignore, and that most of them won't tell you.

Fact No. 1: *A temperature of 98.6 degrees Fahrenheit is not the "normal" temperature for everyone.*

That's what most of us have been told all of our lives, but it simply isn't true. The 98.6-degree standard for body temperature is merely a statistical average, and "normal" for most people is either higher or lower than that. This is particularly true of children. Their "normal" temperatures, measured in carefully controlled studies, ranged from a low of 96.6 degrees to a high of 99.4. Very few of these healthy children registered temperatures of precisely 98.6 degrees.

Your child's temperature may also fluctuate significantly throughout the day. You can expect his temperature to be about a degree higher in the late afternoon than it is in the early morning. Thus, an elevated reading taken at dinnertime may be a perfectly normal reading that occurs at that hour almost every day.

Fact No. 2: *Your child's temperature may rise for a variety of reasons that do not signify illness.*

Children's temperatures may be elevated while they are digesting a heavy meal. They may increase because of ovulation in pubertal teenagers. Sometimes they are a side effect of medications prescribed by your doctor—antihistamines and others.

Fact No. 3: *The fevers you should be concerned about usually stem from an obvious cause.*

Most of the fevers that spell serious trouble are the result of poisoning, or exposure to toxic substances in the environment, and to causes that lead to "heatstroke." You've probably witnessed the latter in person or on TV—the soldier collapsing on the parade ground, or the marathon runner falling by the wayside, because of excessive physical exertion in the hot sun. Temperatures of 107 degrees or above, resulting from these causes, can result in lasting bodily harm, as can those that occur when someone becomes overheated from spending too much time in a sauna or Jacuzzi.

If you suspect that your child has swallowed a poisonous substance, call the poison center immediately. If you can't reach a poison center, don't wait to see if there are adverse reactions. Rush him to a hospital emergency room right away and, if possible, take the poison container with you. That will help determine the appropriate antidote. Most of the time the swallowed substance will be relatively innocuous, but you'll be glad you sought help promptly on the occasion when it isn't.

Immediate treatment is also essential if your child collapses and lapses into unconsciousness—even briefly—after strenuous activity in the hot sun or overexposure in a sauna or a Jacuzzi. Don't just call your doctor. Take the child to a hospital emergency room at once. These external influences are potentially dangerous because they may overwhelm the bodily defenses that normally prevent temperatures from soaring to dangerous levels.

Temperature elevations caused by events of this sort are very rare, of course. They can be identified by your knowledge of the circumstances and the associated symptoms such as loss of consciousness that leave no doubt that your child is in real trouble.

Fact No. 4: *Temperature readings will vary depending on how they are taken.*

Rectal temperatures in older children are usually about a degree higher than those taken orally, and axillary (underarm) temperatures may be about a degree lower. However, in babies rectal temperatures usually vary only slightly from oral or axillary temperatures. Consequently, an axillary reading is quite adequate to determine the temperature of an infant, and the use of a rectal thermometer is unnecessary. Avoid using one and spare your child the hazard of a rectal perforation—a rare accident that sometimes occurs when a rectal thermometer is inserted. I mention this risk only because rectal perforations are fatal in about half the instances in which they occur. That's why I advise parents not to take rectal temperatures. There's no need to do it, so why risk damaging your child?

Finally, don't assume that you can determine the height of fever by placing your hand on your child's chest or forehead. It has been demonstrated that skilled health professionals can't do that with any degree of reliability, and neither can parents.

Fact No. 5: *In advising against the treatment of fever, per se, I make an exception of newborn babies.*

Newborn babies may suffer from infections related to obstetrical intervention during the delivery process, prenatal or hereditary conditions, or events that occur shortly after birth. They may develop scalp abscesses as a result of fetal monitoring prior to delivery or aspiration pneumonia from amniotic fluid forced into the lungs because of overmedication of the mother during labor. They may contact an infection from circumcision performed by the obstetrician before they left the hospital. Finally, they may develop infections from the legion of germs that abound in the hospital itself. (That's one of the reasons all of my grandchildren have been born at home!) Prudence demands that you take your newborn baby to the doctor if he runs a fever of any level during the first few months of life.

Fact No. 6: *If your baby has a fever, don't overlook overdressing as a possible cause.*

Parents, particularly those who are caring for their first child are often overly concerned about keeping the baby warm. They bundle the child up in layer upon layer of clothing and blankets, forgetting that babies are incapable of casting off excess clothing and blankets if the heat becomes oppressive. An elevated temperature may result. If your baby already has a temperature, perhaps accompanied by chills, and you respond by wrapping him tightly in heavy blankets, you will simply force his temperature to rise even more. A simple rule to follow, which I suggest to my patients, is to dress your baby in as many layers of clothing as you find comfortable for yourself.

Fact No. 7: *Most fevers are caused by viral and bacterial infections that the body's own defense mechanisms will overcome without medical help.*

The common cold and influenza are the most common sources of elevated body temperatures in children of all ages. They can generate fevers that range all the way up to 105 degrees, but even at that level they are not a legitimate cause for alarm. The only potential risk is dehydration, which may result from accompanying conditions such as excessive perspiration, rapid respiration, coughing, runny nose, vomiting, and diarrhea. You can help avert the threat of dehydration by making sure that your child receives plenty of fluids. A good rule of thumb is to try to get the patient to drink eight ounces of fluid every hour, preferably liquids that have some nutritional value. However, that's a lot of fluid, and it doesn't make any difference what kind it is, so give your child fruit juice, soda, tea, or anything else he's willing to take.

In most cases you will be able to identify a fever as the product of a viral or bacterial infection, because the accompanying symptoms are those that are typical of these ailments—a mild cough, a stuffy or runny nose, watery eyes, etc. There is no need to call the doctor or to give any form of medication if no other symptoms are present, because there is nothing he or you can prescribe that will cure a viral infection or dispose of a bacterial infection any more effectively than the body's own defenses will. Medications given to relieve discomfort may interfere with the body's efforts to cure itself, for reasons that I'll explore more fully in a later chapter. Antibiotics may shorten the course of a bacterial infection, but the risks outweight the benefit.

Fact No. 8: *There is no consistent relationship between the height of a child's temperature and the severity of a disease.*

There is a common misconception that the height of body temperature is an indication of the severity of an illness, but no consensus exists among parents or even among doctors about what "high" is. I've found among my patients an astonishing range of beliefs on this matter and also about the level a fever must reach before it is "too high." Research has shown that more than half of all parents consider a fever "high" at levels between 100 and 102, and almost all believe it is "high" if it reaches 103 degrees. These parents are also convinced that the height of a fever indicates how sick their child is.

This is emphatically not the case. Knowing the precise level of your child's fever will tell you nothing about how sick he is if the fever is produced by a viral or bacterial infection. Once you have determined that your child has a fever caused by infection, it is useless to hover over him, taking his temperature every hour or so, to determine how high it goes. There is nothing to be gained by measuring its climb, and doing so will probably magnify your fears and upset the child.

Some common, nonthreatening diseases such as roseola (one-day measles) produce extremely high temperatures in some children, while other more serious diseases may not produce any temperature elevation at all. Unless your child's fever is accompanied by additional symptoms, such as vomiting or respiratory difficulties, it need not be a cause of concern, even if it reaches 105.

More important in determining whether a fever is the result of a mild infection like the common cold, or a more serious one such as meningitis, is the overall appearance, behavior, and attitude of your child. These are all factors that you can judge more accurately and skillfully than your doctor, because you are the leading authority on the appearance and behavior of your child. If he is listless or confused, or displays other disturbingly abnormal behavior, a call to your doctor may be warranted if the symptoms persist for a day or two. However, if he's active and playing and behaving normally, you needn't fear that his ailment is a matter of serious concern.

Every now and then I see an article in one of the pediatric journals about "fever phobia." That's a term used by doctors to describe the "unreasonable" fear that some parents have of fever. This is typical of the "blame the victim" attitude that prevails in my profession. Doctors don't make mistakes; when they occur they are always the patient's fault. As far as I'm concerned, "fever phobia" is a disease of pediatricians, not parents, and to the extent that parents are victimized by it, doctors are at fault.

Fact No. 9: *Untreated fevers caused by viral and bacterial infections do not rise inexorably and will not exceed 105 degrees.*

Doctors do a great disservice to you and your child when they prescribe drugs to reduce his fever. The effect of this advice is to validate the common fear of many parents that their child's temperature will continue to rise unless measures are taken to control it and bring it down. They don't tell you that reducing his temperature will do nothing to make the patient well or that our bodies have a built-in mechanism, not fully explained, that will prevent an infection-induced temperature from reaching 106 degrees.

Only in the case of heatstroke, poisoning, or other externally caused fevers is this bodily mechanism over-whelmed and inoperative. It is in those cases that tem-peratures reach and exceed 106 degrees. Doctors know this, but most of them behave as though they didn't. I believe that they are motivated by a simple desire to make you, the parent, believe they have done something to help your child. In addition, they are exhibiting their compulsion to intervene whenever they are provided the opportunity and their reluctance to admit that there are diseases that they can't effectively treat.

Apart from terminal illness, did any doctor *ever* tell a patient, "There's nothing I can do"?

Fact No. 10: *Measures to reduce temperature, such as drugs or sponging, are worse than unnecessary; they are actually counterproductive.*

If your child contracts an infection, the fever that ac-companies it is a blessing, not a curse. It occurs because of the spontaneous release of pyrogens that cause the body temperature to rise. This is a natural defense mech-anism that our bodies employ to fight disease. The pres-ence of fever tells you that the repair mechanisms of the body have gone into high gear.

The process works like this: When an infection de-velops, your child's body responds by manufacturing ad-ditional white blood cells, called *leucocytes*. They destroy bacteria and viruses and remove damaged tissue and irritating materials from the body. The activity of the white cells is also increased, and they move more rapidly to the site of the infection. This part of the process, called *leucotaxis*, is stimulated by the release of the pyrogens that raise body temperature. Hence the fever. A rising body temperature simply indicates that the process of healing is speeding up. It is something to rejoice over, not to fear.

But that isn't all that's happening. Iron, which many germs need in order to thrive, is being removed from the blood and stored in the liver. This reduces the rate at which the bacteria multiply. The action of interferon, a disease-fighting substance produced naturally in the body, also becomes more effective.

Artificially induced fevers have been used in laboratory experiments with animals to demonstrate this process. Elevated temperatures decrease the death rate among animals infected with disease, but if their body temperatures are lowered, more of them die. Artificially induced temperatures have actually been used for many years to treat diseases in humans that do not normally produce fevers themselves.

If your child has a fever resulting from infection, resist the temptation to use drugs or sponging to bring it down. Let the fever run its course. If parental sympathy impels you to do something to relieve your child's discomfort, sponge him off with tepid water or give him one tablet of acetaminophen of the strength recommended for his age. Do nothing beyond that unless the fever persists for more than three days, or other symptoms develop, or your child looks and acts really sick. In that event, see your doctor.

I want to emphasize that, while reducing his fever may make your child more comfortable, you may interfere with the natural healing process if you do it. My only reason for discussing methods of temperature reduction is the probability that some parents won't be able to resist doing it. If you are going to do it, sponging is preferable to drugs because of the risks associated with aspirin and acetaminophen. Despite the frequency of their use, these are far from innocuous drugs. Aspirin probably poisons more children every year than any other toxic substance. It is a form of salicylic acid, which is also the basis for an anticoagulant used in a commercial rat poisons that causes rats to die of internal hemorrhage.

Aspirin can produce a variety of side effects in children and adults, not the least of which is intestinal bleeding. It also has been associated with Reye's syndrome when given to children with influenza or chicken pox. This is an often fatal disease of children primarily affecting the brain and liver. That's one reason so many doctors have switched to prescribing acetaminophen (Tylenol, etc.). That doesn't really solve the problem, because evidence is emerging that large doses of this drug may be toxic to the liver and kidneys. It is also worth noting that babies born to mothers who take aspirin near the end of labor or during delivery sometimes are victims of cephalhematoma, a condition in which fluid-filled bumps appear on the scalp.

If you can't resist sponging your child to bring down his fever, use tepid water, not cold water or alcohol. The reduction of fever by sponging is caused by evaporation, not by the temperature of the water. There is no added benefit in sponging your child with water that is uncomfortably cold. Don't use alcohol, because it is no more effective than tepid water, and the fumes released on evaporation may be toxic to a small child.

Fact No. 11: *Fevers produced by viral or bacterial infections will not cause brain damage or permanent physical harm.*

The fear of fevers in the higher ranges stems primarily from the widespread belief that permanent physical or brain damage may result if you permit your child's fever to get "too high." If that were true, it would justify any level of panic a parent might display, and because many parents believe it is true, it often does.

If you have harbored this fear, put aside everything you have been led to believe about fever by your doctor, your parents, your grandparents, your spouse, or even the friendly medical expert who lives next door and offers her advice over your morning cup of coffee. Even grandmothers are not always right! Your child's cold, influenza, or any other infection will not produce a fever that exceeds 106 degrees, and below that level the fever will not cause any lasting harm.

Because your child's bodily defenses won't allow infections to produce fevers of 106 degrees, you need not live in fear of mental or physical damage when his temperature begins to rise. I doubt that many pediatricians, including those who have practiced for decades, have seen more than one or two cases of fever above 106 degrees during their entire careers. Those they did see were the result of causes other than infection, such as poisoning or heatstroke. I have treated tens of thousands of children, and I've seen only one case of fever higher than 106. That's not surprising, because it is estimated that 95 percent of childhood fevers don't even reach 105.

Fact No. 12: *High fevers do not cause convulsions. They result when the temperature rises at an extremely rapid rate.*

Many parents are fearful of fevers because they have witnessed a convulsive seizure and believe that their child may experience one if his temperature is allowed to rise "too high." I empathize with those who have this concern, for a child in the throes of a convulsion is a frightening spectacle. If you have seen one occur, you may find it hard to believe that this condition is rarely serious. It is also relatively uncommon; it is estimated that only 4 percent of children with high fever experience fever-related convulsions. There is no evidence that those who do have them suffer any serious aftereffects as a result. One study of 1,706 children who had suffered febrile convulsions failed to disclose a single death or motor defect. There is also no convincing evidence that febrile seizures in childhood increase susceptibility to epilepsy later in life.

More to the point, however, is the fact that treatment to prevent febrile convulsions is almost always given too late to do any good. Medication and sponging are a useless exercise because, by the time you become aware that your child has a temperature, the probability is that any resulting convulsion would already have occurred. That's because the convulsion is not related to the height of your child's temperature but to how rapidly the temperature rose to whatever level it reached. By the time you become aware of the child's temperature, the probability is that this rapid rise has already occurred, and unless the child has already convulsed, the danger period has passed.

The possibility of febrile convulsions is limited primarily to children under five years of age, and even those children who experience them prior to that age rarely have them after the age of five. When a child experiences a convulsion, many doctors will prescribe long-term therapy with phenobarbital or other anticonvulsants to prevent a recurrence of seizures when another fever occurs.

If your doctor suggests this treatment for your child, I urge you to question him about the risks of long-term anticonvulsant therapy. Also ask him about the behavioral changes it may produce in your child. There is no consensus among doctors on the long-term management of febrile seizures. The drugs commonly used can cause liver damage, and animal studies suggest that they may have a negative impact on the development of the brain. One authority on the subject has argued that "Some patients may be better off leading a more normal life between occasional seizures than they would if they lived seizure-free in a perpetual state of drug-induced drowsiness and confusion. . . ."

I was trained to prescribe phenobarbital for children who had febrile convulsions, in order to prevent recurrences. The same treatment strategy is still being taught to students in medical school. I began to develop doubts about this procedure when I saw that some patients had repeat convulsions even when they were taking phenobarbital. That obviously raised a question about whether those who were taking phenobarbital and were seizure-free were benefiting from the drug or would have escaped another convulsion even if they hadn't used it. My doubts were enhanced when some mothers began to report that phenobarbital overstimulated their children instead of quieting them or quieted them so much that normally active, outgoing kids became, by comparison, semizombies. Because convulsions are so infrequent, and cause no lasting damage, I no longer prescribe this therapy for the children who are entrusted to my care.

If your child suffers a febrile convulsion and your pediatrician prescribes long-term anticonvulsant therapy, you will have to determine whether you want to accept it. I know it may be difficult for you to question the treatments prescribed by your pediatrician and that when you do you may get a brusque and unresponsive reply. If this is what happens when you question your pediatrician about a medication, there's not much point in arguing with him. Accept the prescription and then get a second opinion from another doctor before you decide whether to have it filled.

If your son or daughter does experience a fever-induced convulsion, try not to panic. That's advice that is far easier for me to give than it may be for you to follow, because the sight of your child in the midst of a convulsion may be so unnerving. Calm yourself by remembering that the convulsions are not life-threatening and will not result in physical damage and then take a few simple steps to protect your child from injury.

First, place the child on his side so that he will not choke on his own saliva. Next, keep him from striking his head against any hard or sharp object while he is thrashing about. Make sure that he does not have a breathing obstruction during the seizure and place some soft but firm object such as a folded leather glove or billfold (not your finger) between his teeth to keep him from biting his tongue. Then, for your own peace of mind, call your doctor and tell him what happened.

Most seizures last no more than a few minutes. If one

is prolonged, call your doctor and ask for his advice. You may expect the child to sleep after the seizure has passed, but even if he doesn't, don't give him anything to eat or drink for an hour or so. He may be so drowsy that he aspirates the food and chokes on it.

DR. MENDELSOHN'S QUICK REFERENCE GUIDE TO FEVER

Fevers are a common symptom in children and are not an indication of serious illness unless associated with major changes in appearance and behavior or other major symptoms such as respiratory difficulty or loss of consciousness. The height of fever is not a measure of the severity of an illness. Infection-induced fevers will not reach levels that can cause permanent damage to your child. Fevers do not usually require medical attention, except as recommended below. They are the body's natural defense against infection and should be allowed to run their course without medication or other treatment intended to bring them down.

1. If your child is less than two months of age, and his temperature exceeds 100 degrees, call your doctor. The fever may be the symptom of an infection that is prenatal in origin or related to the delivery of the baby. Fevers in newborn infants are so uncommon that simple prudence and your peace of mind make a visit to the doctor worthwhile, even though it may prove to be unnecessary.

2. For older children it is unnecessary to call the doctor unless the fever fails to abate within three days or is accompanied by other major symptoms such as vomiting, respiratory distress, persistent cough lasting several days, and other major symptoms not normally associated

with the common cold. Also see your doctor if your child displays continued listlessness, irritability, inattentiveness, or otherwise acts and looks seriously ill.

3. Call your doctor, regardless of the temperature level, if your child is experiencing difficulty in breathing, is vomiting repeatedly, or has a fever that is accompanied by twitching or other strange movements, or you are concerned about any other alarming element of the child's behavior or appearance.

4. If your child experiences chills along with his fever, don't try to counteract it by piling on more blankets. This will simply cause the temperature to increase more rapidly, and the chills are not to be feared, because they are a normal bodily response. The chills do not mean that the child is cold but are part of the mechanism through which the body adjusts to a higher temperature level.

5. Encourage your feverish child to rest, but don't make too big a production of it. There is no medical need to confine him to bed or even to keep him indoors if the weather is reasonably decent. The fresh air and moderate activity may improve his disposition and make him easier to live with, and it won't make him any sicker. You should try to discourage him from engaging in intense competitive sports, however.

6. If you have reason to believe that the fever is the result of a cause other than infection, such as heatstroke or poisoning, take your child to a hospital emergency room at once. If there is no emergency room in your area, seek medical attention wherever it is available.

7. Ignore the old wives' tale "Feed a cold and starve a fever." Nourishment is an important

part of recovery from any illness. To the extent your child will tolerate it, you should feed both colds and fevers. Both conditions burn up the body's supply of protein, fats, and carbohydrates, and they should be replaced. If the child won't eat, give him fluids such as fruit juice that have some caloric value. And don't forget, you don't have to be Jewish to benefit from chicken soup!

8. Fevers and the other symptoms commonly associated with it may cause your child to lose a significant volume of fluids. This could lead to dehydration, but you can help avert it by making sure that he drinks plenty of fluids. Fruit juices are fine, but if he resists them, almost any other fluid will do. The trick is to try to get him to consume eight ounces an hour.

8

Headache: *Usually Emotional, but the Pain Is Real*

Almost every abnormal condition of the body—organic, psychological, or emotional—can cause a headache. The most common organic cause in children is viral or bacterial infection anywhere in the body, but allergies, metabolic disturbances, or trauma may also be responsible. The next most frequent cause is psychological or emotional stress.

Headaches rarely require medical treatment, and when they do it is treatment of the disease or injury that is causing the headache, not treatment of the headache itself. The immediate need, when your child says his "head hurts," is to identify the cause. In most instances you can do this as readily, and perhaps more effectively, than your doctor.

Doctors take a statistical approach in their search for the cause of a headache. They attempt, by questioning the child and his parents, to determine whether any other symptoms are present or whether any unusual events have occurred prior to its onset that may be an emotional source of the headache. If this is unproductive, and no clinical findings emerge from a physical examination, the doctor will perform a series of inclusionary and exclusionary tests, searching for some possible causes and excluding others. Based on the statistical frequency of the possible causes, he will begin a process of elimination. If this fails to yield a positive finding, he will probably assume that the headache is the result of some form of emotional or psychological stress. He will then probably prescribe an analgesic preparation, such as acetaminophen (Tylenol) or aspirin. He will also caution the parents to observe the child closely in order to detect the possible emergence of additional symptoms.

My experience has taught me that 85–90 percent of childhood headaches can be diagnosed on the basis of history alone. It doesn't require a visit to the doctor to determine whether your child has a cold or the flu or suffered an emotional upset prior to the onset of the headache. Most of the time you are far more capable of identifying the cause than your doctor is. You alone have the opportunity to monitor your child's behavior and reactions around the clock in a search for the conditions or events that may be provoking the psychological or emotional trauma. You are familiar with the child's normal behavior patterns, and in most cases you ultimately will sense what is bothering him. In short, you have the knowledge and the experience to isolate a psychological or emotional cause, and your doctor doesn't. All he has to go on is the minimal amount of information he can extract from you or your child during a brief office visit.

That's why, if your child has a headache, it is premature to rush him to a doctor immediately. Before you do you should begin a structured program of observation and questioning to attempt to identify the cause. Also, if your child is very young, be sure that when he says his "head hurts" he really means a headache. You wouldn't believe the number of children who have been brought to me for treatment of headaches who were really complaining about external pain they felt because their sister or a playmate socked him with a toy!

HOW TO DISCOVER THE CAUSE OF HEADACHES

Begin your investigation by exploring the basic areas that are most often the source of childhood headache pain. Determine the answers to these questions:

1. Does your child also have the symptoms of a common cold or influenza that are described in Chapter 10? If so, you can safely assume that the headache is an additional symptom of one of those ailments and requires no medical treatment.

2. Did the child experience a fall or blow on the head prior to the onset of the headache? Was this traumatic event accompanied by loss of consciousness? If so, or if there are other disturbing symptoms such as disorientation or dizziness, call your doctor or, better still, take the child to a hospital emergency room. If the injury occurred outside your presence, and you are unable to determine whether there was loss of consciousness, play it safe and call your doctor.

3. Has there been a recent change in your child's diet that might signify an allergy to foods he has not eaten before? Has your family moved to a new location where there are types of vegetation that your child has not been exposed to before?

4. When did you first notice the headaches? Was the initial one preceded by some unpleasant, frightening, or otherwise emotionally traumatic event?

5. Do the headaches typically recur at the same time each day? Does this indicate association

with anticipation of some specific event or activity—school, piano lessons, etc.?

6. Is the child closely associated with another person who routinely uses headaches to get attention or sympathy or to evade responsibility?

7. What unpleasant or tiresome work, or threatening events or activities, has the child avoided because of previous headaches?

8. What rewards has the child obtained from previous headaches? Don't overlook increased attention and sympathy.

Within these broad categories some specific potential causes of the headaches may emerge in response to these additional questions:

- Has your child had a recent emotional upset because of some circumstance involving family or friends? (Examples: the death of a loved one; a parental dispute that may have raised concern about the possibility of a divorce or separation.)

- Could the headache be prompted by an unpleasant or frightening situation? (Examples: fear of a physical encounter with a schoolmate; fear of a reprimand at school for undone homework; concern about a scheduled test.)

- Could the headache be the result of some recent change in normal life patterns? (Examples: separation from friends or relatives; a move to a new home and the need to make new friends; an ailment contracted on a vacation trip; the onset of the heating season.)

- Could the headache be prompted by a desire to escape responsibility? Did the child "borrow" the symptom from a relative or other close associate who routinely uses headaches as a means of avoiding work or responsibility? (Example: if your child is compelled to do the dishes alone because Aunt Mabel always gets a headache just before it's time to do them, he may get the message!)

- What events are immediately associated with the onset of the headaches and with their disappearance? (Example: suspect problems with friends or teachers at school if the child complains of a headache while at the breakfast table, but it disappears soon after you agree to let him stay home from school.)

EVEN EMOTIONAL HEADACHES ARE REAL

Always bear in mind that, although your child's headache may be emotional rather than organic in origin, it is nonetheless real. The common adult protest, "You give me a headache," is often more than an expression of annoyance. The behavior of others, worry, fear, anger—the whole range of human emotions—can, at one time or another, literally give you, and your child as well, an honest-to-goodness headache that really hurts.

If you identify a cause of this nature, the treatment should not be medical. It requires the practice of sound, sympathetic parenting. The child needs your help, displayed through love, affection, understanding, moral support, and a demonstration of genuine parental concern. Giving the child an analgesic such as aspirin or Tylenol is not a substitute for the emotional support that he needs.

In most cases patient observation and a review of recent events and conditions will identify the cause of the headache. If those measures fail, continue to observe the child closely to detect any additional symptoms that may develop. These might include fever, vomiting, coughing, skin rashes, visual disturbances, weight loss, chronic fatigue and lassitude, and any other physical variations from the child's normal condition.

The location of the headache may also be helpful in determining the cause. If the pain is in the front of the head, suspect the sinuses as the source of the trouble. An additional indication would be a greenish or yellow discharge from the nose. This condition will usually cure itself, and limited amounts of Tylenol can be used appropriately to relieve the pain if it becomes unbearable. Meanwhile, use a vaporizer to help relieve the condition by opening up the nasal passages to permit drainage and give your child ample fluids to prevent dehydration. If these measures fail, and the headache pain becomes unbearable, you may be compelled to take your child to a doctor to obtain a prescription for a more effective pain reliever—codeine. I don't like to prescribe this drug, or any other narcotic, because it is addictive and has many possible side effects, some of them serious. However, limited use of codeine for the relief of acute pain is acceptable.

If sinus attacks recur, it is time to look to prevention rather than repeated treatment. Consider the possibility of food or environmental allergies as the cause and begin an attempt to identify the offending substance or substances yourself or obtain the help of a competent specialist. Dr. Theron Randolph, of Chicago, author of the excellent book, *Alternative Approaches to Allergy*, heads a group called the Human Ecology Action League, which maintains a register of specialists in this field. You can write him at P.O. Box 1369, Evanston, IL 60204, or telephone him at (312) 864-0995, for the name of a practitioner in your area.

Note that the frontal sinuses do not develop until the age of six, so if your child is younger than that, a sinus infection is not apt to be the problem. Another word of caution: Sinus problems can be magnified by changes in air pressure, so do not take your child in an airplane when he is suffering from this condition.

HEADACHES RESULTING FROM TENSION

Pain in the back of the head is more likely to be a product of tension that is of emotional origin. If the pain is on the side of the head, there is the possibility that it may be migraine, although this is rare in children and virtually unknown prior to the age of 10. Migraine headaches are usually familial or hereditary, but allergic causes should also be sought. They are frequently associated with vomiting and disappear after the victim has vomited and goes to sleep. There is no specific treatment, other than the use of analgesics to relieve the pain.

If all of your careful probing fails to reveal the source of the headaches, and they continue to plague your child, it is appropriate to seek the help of a doctor. Your time and effort have not been wasted, however, because you will be able to provide detailed information that will assist him in making an accurate diagnosis. It is also appropriate to see a doctor, of course, if associated symptoms develop that cannot be related to the onset of a cold, influenza, or some other common ailment.

When you see your doctor, share with him fully what you have learned in your own search for a possible cause because all of this information is an essential part of the careful history he should take. If he seems uninterested, and unwilling to spend the time required, you may have the wrong doctor.

Your doctor should also do a careful and thorough physical examination, which usually proceeds from head to toe. It should include these elements:

- *Examination of the back of the eye with an ophthalmoscope, which reveals the condition of the retina.* By looking at the nerves and blood vessels at the back of the eye the doctor can discover abnormalities that may indicate vascular disorders or increased intracranial pressure, which might be caused by a brain tumor. Such tumors are extremely rare in children and, if present, are also revealed by vomiting and nausea, which is often more noticeable in the early morning; fainting spells; dizziness; vision problems; and other neurological abnormalities. Brain tumors in children are so uncommon that they rank far down on the list of probable headache causes.

- *Examination of the eardrums and external air canal with an otoscope, which enables the doctor to observe eardrum perforations, infection, or the presence of a foreign body.* Small children may put crayons, beans, beads, and other objects in their ears, which may become infected and cause a headache.

- *Measurement of blood pressure with a small cuff that is appropriate for the size of the child.* High blood pressure can indicate kidney problems, certain tumors, and vascular malfunctions.

- *A careful neurological examination, during which the doctors tests your child's reflexes with a reflex hammer and his sensory functions with pins, brushes, and a tuning fork.* The doctor is looking for the presence of tendon and other reflexes that normally are equal in both extremities. The absence of uniform reflexes in both arms and legs may indicate an abnormality of the central or peripheral nervous system, spinal cord diseases, the possibility of a brain tumor, and other neurologic malfunctions.

- *A stethoscopic examination of the heart and chest and—equally important—the pulses in various parts of the body.* This will detect heart ailments, lung problems, and vascular disorders.

- *A completely stripped physical examination should be performed during which the doctor visually inspects every part of your child's body, although not necessarily all at once.* He should

check the abdomen to determine abnormalities of
the liver, the thyroid gland, and the lymph nodes.

The sort of examination I have just described is what
your sick child deserves but doesn't always get. Pediatricians typically schedule so many patients that they tend
to rush through everything, including history taking and
physical examinations. In fact, many doctors are careless in the conduct of physical examinations. I first observed this while I was an intern at Cook County
Hospital in Chicago. Examinations were given there for
prospective board specialists, and as part of the exam
the candidate was presented with a patient who was in
bed, under the covers. Not infrequently, the candidate
who conducted the examination failed to discover that
the patient had a wooden leg! While working in the
emergency room in the same hospital I received a patient
from the Michael Reese emergency room who brought
with him a note containing the diagnosis—a coronary
heart attack. When I removed his jacket I found a stab
wound!

DON'T BE AFRAID TO QUESTION
YOUR DOCTOR

So, don't assume that your doctor will do a thorough
physical examination, and if he fails to do one, question
him about it. If your question makes him angry, or he
brushes you off with an evasive answer, consider finding
another doctor. If you feel the need to give him a reason
for your question, tell him what you read in this book.
That *will* make him angry!

If the doctor fails to elicit a cause for the headaches
from the history and the physical findings—and maybe
even if he does—he will probably tell you he is going to
perform some tests. These should include a blood test
and a urinalysis, to reveal hidden infections and metabolic disorders such as diabetes. I approve of both of

these tests, if another cause for the headache has not been found, because—unlike many of the tests that doctors routinely use—they provide a high degree of valid answers. However, I have some strong reservations about how far beyond these two tests a doctor should go.

For example, taking an X-ray of the skull, or a CAT scan, or performing an electroencephalogram (EEG), is rarely productive, but many doctors are fond of ordering them. That's because too many doctors seem to believe that anything they *can* do they *must* do. In my judgment, skull X-rays and CAT scans are rarely indicated and usually should be avoided, as should all needless exposure to radiation. Even a history of a traumatic head injury is not an indication for skull X-ray, unless the injury was accompanied by a period of unconsciousness following the injury, persistent vomiting, or other symptoms such as inability to focus the eyes or loss of memory.

The same warning applies to the EEG, a procedure that is valuable in detecting the presence of brain tumors and blood clots and diagnosing epilepsy but is unreliable for most other purposes. As a diagnostic tool, in general, the answers that it provides are as likely to be wrong as they are to be right. Studies have shown that 20 percent of the patients with serious and life-threatening neurological problems show normal EEGs, and 20 percent of the patients with no neurologic problems have "abnormal" readings. In one of my earlier books I reported the experience of one researcher who connected an EEG machine to a mannequin that had a head stuffed with lime gelatin. The machine pronounced the mannequin to be alive and well!

When he has completed his examination, your doctor may recommend the use of drugs. Limited use of an analgesic is appropriate for the relief of pain *if the cause of the headache has been determined* but to be avoided if it has not, because of the risks associated with both aspirin and acetaminophen. Reject the use of antihistamines and psychotropic drugs unless a firm diagnosis has been made and the doctor can defend their use. You have every right, although he may not like it, to question your doctor about the potential benefits of any drug he prescribes and about how those benefits stack up against the potential risks and side effects of the drug.

My objection to the use of drugs for the relief of headache pain if no cause of the headache has been found deserves further explanation. Pain is nature's way of signaling that something is wrong. The use of analgesics may end the pain, but it doesn't solve the underlying problem. Your child is still sick, but if the pain is gone, there is less incentive to continue to search for the condition that caused it. It is important that you and your doctor be alert for the emergence of additional symptoms until the headaches disappear without the use of drugs or their cause is identified.

Here is my advice to parents whose child has recurrent headaches:

DR. MENDELSOHN'S QUICK REFERENCE GUIDE TO HEADACHES

1. Avoid emotionally triggered childhood headaches by providing a warm, sensitive, caring, loving environment for your child. Try to establish a confiding relationship with him, so that you can provide moral support and comfort when there are events or situations in his life that are disturbing to him. Never forget, for a moment, that this is the parents' primary role and the one that will have the greatest impact on the health and development of your child.

2. Be careful not to impose excessive demands on your child that will cause him to become emotionally ill because of his fear that he cannot live up to your expectations. Children cannot and should not be expected to assume the burdens of adults for, as someone else has

said, "the business of a child is to play and to learn."

3. If your child complains of recurrent headaches and no other symptoms are present, attempt to determine the cause yourself. Eliminate emotional causes and the onset of a common cold or influenza as possibilities before you turn to other potential causes.

4. Unless other symptoms are present, there is no immediate need for concern that the headache may indicate more serious physical problems. A call or visit to the doctor is premature.

5. If your anxiety level becomes too high, and your child's headache is giving *you* one, take him to the doctor but monitor carefully what he does to the child.

6. If the headache becomes incessant, or recurs throughout the day for several days, see your doctor even though there are no other symptoms.

7. When you do visit a physician, be sure he takes a careful history, in addition to conducting a thorough physical and neurological examination. Your child is deserving of the best your doctor has to offer, and if he doesn't get it, consider finding another doctor.

8. Question any tests the doctor wants to conduct, other than a blood count and a urinalysis. Resist other tests, such as skull x-rays and EEGs, unless associated symptoms are present or abnormal findings were discovered during the physical and neurological exams. Demand an explanation of the need for any additional tests the doctor wants to do. If this angers the doctor, or he is evasive, consider finding another doctor.

9. Reject all medication except mild analgesics for short-term relief of pain, unless it can be defended as a specific for a known cause of the headaches. Don't accept "just-in-case" medication. Meanwhile, insist that the doctor continue to monitor the physical and neurological condition of your child while you remain alert for the development of additional symptoms that may help pinpoint the cause.

10. If you know that the headache was caused by an accidental injury, and there was loss of consciousness or your child is dizzy, disoriented, or confused, take him to a hospital emergency room. Do this also if the injury occurred outside your presence and you cannot determine whether he experienced a period of unconsciousness.

9

Mother, My Tummy Hurts!

A bdominal pain ranks with fever and the common cold as a leading source of pointless visits to pediatricians. It is a common phenomenon in children, but the pain rarely stems from organic causes, so it usually does not indicate a serious illness. I estimate, in my own practice, that only one in 10 of the children brought to me because of "stomachaches" actually needs medical attention.

Unless abdominal pain is accompanied by other symptoms—notably vomiting, diarrhea, loss of appetite, and weight loss—it is usually nothing you need to worry about. A bit of careful detective work on your part will probably isolate a nonmedical cause for your child's discomfort. In most cases you will discover that your child's frequent belly pains are the result of indigestion from eating too much or too fast; are the by-product of another ailment; are the result of psychological or emotional causes; or are produced by allergies to food, medications, or chemical additives to the food that he eats.

The psychological and emotional causes parallel those already described for headaches. Let's say, for example, that your child repeatedly develops abdominal pain in the morning, just before it is time to go to school. You are reluctant to have him miss his classes, but he appears to be in such agony that you finally agree to let him stay home from school. In all probability he will experience a miraculous recovery the moment the school bus disappears down the street!

After this scene has been repeated a few times you may be tempted to reprimand or punish your child for deceiving you. Don't, because the pain was real, but it disappeared promptly—as it should have—when the trauma that caused it was relieved.

This reaction is so common that it even has a name— *school phobia*—and you can't solve the problem by taking your child to a doctor. Instead, his pain is your cue to undertake some patient and sympathetic interrogation to determine the association between his school and his pain. Is he being bullied while waiting for the school bus or after he gets to school? Is he having discipline problems with his teachers? Is he ashamed and worried because he hasn't been completing his homework? Does he have an incompetent teacher he simply can't stand? Or, if he is very young, is he simply troubled over being separated from you and sent off to a strange and possibly frightening environment? If you can identify and eliminate the cause of his concern, it is likely that his pains will be eliminated, too.

As in the case of headaches, stomachaches may evolve as a form of subconscious avoidance of unpleasant tasks or a desire to gain sympathetic attention from parents who are not fully satisfying their child's need to feel loved. A lot of recurrent "tummy aches" would clear up if more parents heeded the advice on the bumper stickers, "Have you hugged your kid today?"

STOMACHACHES OFTEN CAUSED BY ALLERGIES

Allergies to foods and chemicals are another frequent source of belly pain. Lactose intolerance—allergy to cow's milk—is far more common than most parents realize. In addition to milk, however, there is a broad range of foods to which children (and adults) may be allergic.

You can determine whether a food allergy is causing your child's abdominal pain by developing a structured program to determine whether one or more of the foods he eats are consistently associated with his malady. This requires time and effort and may elicit some childish cries of protest, but if food allergies are the problem, it works. Withdraw specific food items from his diet, one by one, and observe whether the recurrent pains disappear after a few days. If this yields a likely suspect, reinstate the food item and see whether the pains recur. If so, you've found the answer!

The process will be more difficult if your child has multiple food allergies, because eliminating one offender may not eliminate the pain, which will still be produced by others. In that event you will have to reverse the process by eliminating all of the most probable allergens from his diet and then restoring them one by one. If the pains recur when a food is added, you will have identified one of the culprits. Eliminate it permanently and then continue to restore other food items, one at a time, until you have identified everything to which he is allergic.

If you use the first approach, you will expedite the process by beginning the elimination process with the most likely candidates. Foods with chemical additives are major offenders, and eliminating them means that you will have to eliminate virtually all processed foods and manufactured products and resort to natural foods, cooked from scratch. Don't overlook breads, pastries, and even pastas. Buy natural foods, products labeled "100-percent natural," and read the labels carefully. Natural foods that are likely offenders include tomatoes, cucumbers, oranges, apricots, prunes, peaches, plums, raspberries, and grapes, but your child may be allergic to others.

Let me warn you that you will be startled to discover how prevalent chemicals are in our daily diets when you begin looking for foods that don't contain them. The fine print on many food packages would ruin the appetites of most consumers if their eyesight were good enough to decipher it. How would you like a nice bowl of soup made from sodium carbonate, potassium carbonate, sodium tripolyphosphate, sodium alginate, disodium phosphate, disodium inosinate, and disodium guanylate? If you were offered it, knowing what it contained, you probably would be afraid to eat it, and you should be. Yet these are all ingredients in one popular brand of Chinese noodle soup mix!

All of the chemical colorings, preservatives, stabilizers, and taste enhancers are potential sources of allergic reactions, to say nothing of more hazardous effects. They are a prime cause of hyperactivity, which I'll discuss in detail later. They are not easy to avoid, but if you can avoid them, the benefits will not be limited to curing your child's abdominal pain. The more you rely on natural foods as the basis of your family fare, the healthier you and everyone else in your household will be.

I urge you to become a food detective for two reasons. First, your doctor couldn't do it if he wanted to, and he doesn't want to. Second, if you are able to identify and eliminate the source of your child's discomfort, you will help him avoid the even greater discomfort and potential risks that may result if you take him to a doctor. If your child has recurrent abdominal pain but is growing well, looks healthy, is gaining height and weight, and has no other symptoms, there is no appropriate medical treatment for the condition and no need to see a doctor. Provide moral support and look for an allergic or emotional cause.

DON'T USE MEDICINE TO "CURE" STOMACHACHES

I don't recommend the use of any medication when your child complains of a "stomachache." Some parents respond by giving their child sodium bicarbonate (baking soda) or one of the over-the-counter antacid preparations. This is unwise for two reasons. First, when your child complains of a "stomachache," the pain he refers to may not be in his stomach but elsewhere in the abdomen —in the intestines, kidneys, or some other organ. In that event the antacid won't provide relief. Second, if he really has pain produced by excess stomach acid, which is unlikely in children, sodium bicarbonate may relieve it temporarily, but because it neutralizes all of the acid in the stomach, it will cause a rebound effect. The child's stomach will work overtime replacing the acid, probably with more acid than was there before. The only sensible immediate relief you can offer is a generous dose of love, comfort, sympathy, and distraction. If the symptom is emotional in origin, that may end the pain.

I do not mean to suggest that abdominal pain is always innocuous. It is *one* symptom of well over 50 diseases, some of them serious and even life-threatening. In every case, however, if it does indicate a serious problem, there are other symptoms as well. The risk, if you take your child to the doctor, is that he will ignore the possibility of a nutritional or emotional cause and begin an ill-advised diagnostic process based on the presence of one symptom alone. Because abdominal pain is one symptom of so many diseases, he has an almost endless array of tests that he may inflict on your child. Many of these tests are only marginally accurate, which may lead to a false diagnosis. Many are painful and needlessly traumatic for your child and, consequently, for you as well. Virtually all of them are dangerous, and some even carry a mortality rate. Yet, without any additional symptoms, none of them is necessary.

A further risk is the possibility that the doctor may hospitalize your child in order to perform these tests. Many of them require advance preparation, such as cleaning out the bowel, which is more readily and thoroughly accomplished if your child is hospitalized. That's a high price to pay, in more ways than money, for what will probably be a fruitless search. In addition to the risks inherent in the tests and X-rays themselves, there is the emotional trauma most children experience when hospitalized. There is also the very real danger that your healthy child will acquire an illness while he is in the hospital.

If your child *does* display a number of symptoms in addition to pain, such as vomiting, diarrhea, or bloody stools, he should be taken to a doctor. As I have indicated previously, he could be the victim of any one of several ailments, the most likely of which is appendicitis.

DIAGNOSIS OF APPENDICITIS

The incidence of appendicitis is highest among males between the ages of 15 and 30 years, but it is found at all ages, even among infants during their first weeks of life. It is perhaps most dangerous among very young children because it is difficult to diagnose, and in a majority of cases the appendix ruptures before the diagnosis is made.

Appendicitis is almost invariably accompanied by vomiting and fever, but the vomiting may not be persistent and the fever may be very mild. In its early stages the pain is usually general throughout the abdomen, but within a matter of hours it localizes in the lower right quadrant, and pressure at that point will cause intense pain. If the appendix subsequently ruptures, the pain will again become generalized throughout the abdominal area. The attack is almost always preceded by a loss of appetite.

When you take your child to the doctor he should take a careful history, with particular attention paid to events that preceded the onset of the pain. He should conduct a thorough physical examination, including exercises that will help identify the site of the pain. These should include asking your child to raise his legs while lying on his back, which puts a strain on the abdominal muscles, and also observing him while he walks to determine whether he is favoring the one side of the abdomen because of pain. A blood test should be taken to determine whether there is an elevated white cell count, indicating infection, and a urinalysis, to reveal the presence of white blood cells, indicating urinary tract infection.

If, as a result of his examination, the pediatrician suspects appendicitis, he will probably refer your child to a surgeon. If the surgeon recommends removal of the appendix, insist that your pediatrician concur in the recommendation and share the responsibility. Surgeons are in the business of doing surgery, and if there is a legitimate reason to suspect appendicitis, they will usually seize the opportunity to put their talents to work. As a consequence, thousands of perfectly healthy appendices are removed every year. That's not only painful and expensive, but there is substantial reason to believe that the appendix performs some useful functions, so it is unwise to allow your child's appendix to be removed unless he is at risk. In addition, while appendicitis can be fatal, particularly if the organ ruptures, appendectomies have a mortality rate of their own which is almost as high as that of appendicitis itself. Be certain that your pediatrician and the surgeon agree on the diagnosis and that there is a significant possibility that the appendix may rupture, before you permit your child to endure the risk of surgery.

If you do agree to surgery, insist that your pediatrician be present in the operating room when the surgery is performed. That's simply insurance against something going wrong, and it also provides you with a witness in case something does. It isn't generally known, but a lot of research takes place in the operating rooms of teaching hospitals, sometimes without the knowledge or consent of the patient or his parents. It is prudent to insist that your pediatrician be present during the surgery to make certain that your child does not become the unwitting subject of a research procedure.

Recurrent abdominal pain can be terribly frustrating,

as can any chronic physical condition that makes your child miserable, because inevitably his misery rubs off on you. Fortunately, to employ a classic medical cop-out, you don't have to "learn to live with it." Follow the guidelines I've given you in this chapter and you should be able to identify the cause of your child's recurrent pain.

DR. MENDELSOHN'S QUICK REFERENCE GUIDE TO ABDOMINAL PAIN

Most childhood abdominal pain does not require medical attention unless it is accompanied by additional symptoms. Consequently, you should make that distinction when your child complains that his "tummy hurts." Here are the guidelines that will enable you to determine whether the cause may be appendicitis, an intestinal obstruction, or another serious ailment that requires the help of a doctor or is a problem you can handle yourself.

1. If abdominal pain is the only symptom, you are more able than your doctor to identify the cause. However, if it is accompanied by additional symptoms such as fever, vomiting, pain on urination, or bloody stools, your doctor should be consulted.

2. If there is no additional symptom, carefully review the events and circumstances that preceded the onset of the abdominal pain. Had your child eaten too much too fast? Had he eaten or drunk anything to which he was unaccustomed? Could he have ingested a poisonous substance or swallowed an object such as a marble or a safety pin? Had he been given some medication he had never taken before? Had he experienced some traumatic event—a fight or

argument with a playmate, a bad report card, a severe reprimand or punishment? If stomach-aches have been a recurrent phenomenon, was each of these preceded by a similar event? Have they been associated with avoidance of an undesirable experience (e.g., school) or unpleasant tasks (e.g., washing dishes)? A painstaking review of this kind should enable you to determine whether the pain is of emotional origin.

3. If a visit to the doctor is indicated, monitor his actions. Make certain that he takes a careful history and conducts a thorough physical examination. This should include a blood test to determine whether there is an elevated white cell count, indicating infection; a urinalysis to determine whether white blood cells are present, indicating a urinary tract infection; and examination to determine whether the pain is localized in the lower right quadrant of the abdomen, indicating appendicitis.

4. If the doctor concludes that your child's appendix is the culprit, he may refer you to a surgeon. If surgery is recommended, insist that your pediatrician concur and share responsibility for that decision. Then, insist that he be present in the operating room when the operation is performed.

5. Don't leave your child alone in the hospital before or after the surgery is performed. Remain with him yourself or have a friend or relative do so until you are sure he is well on the road to recovery. Then get him released from the hospital as soon as you possibly can.

10

Coughs, Sneezes, and Runny Noses

Americans spend more each year on over-the-counter remedies for coughs and colds than the combined costs of running the governments of Guatemala, Honduras, and El Salvador. If you added what's spent for antibiotics, antihistamines, and other medications prescribed by doctors, you could probably throw in Costa Rica and Ecuador, too. That's an appropriate comparison, because most of those governments don't work very well, and the cold medicines don't work, either.

Coughs, colds, and influenza affect all of us, but children seem to be more susceptible to them than adults and more likely to be treated for them when they occur. While the treatment may relieve cold symptoms, none of the drugs that are given will effect a cure. In fact, needless and often counterproductive medication has given rise to a private joke among doctors that is not shared with patients: without treatment a common cold usually lasts about seven days; with treatment it will last about a week.

The common cold is such a universal phenomenon, affecting almost everyone at least once during the year, that theories abound about its causes and how it should be treated. These theories can be divided roughly into two categories—the moral theory and the viral theory. The moral theory, based on the higher incidence of colds in winter, holds that they are related to exposure to inclement weather. This theory, a favorite of mothers and grandmothers, argues that a child caught a cold because he didn't put on his muffler, mittens, or galoshes. The viral theory, espoused by doctors, says that colds are caused by one of 100 or more viruses and that they occur more frequently in winter because children are in school and are exposed to infected children in the confinement of the classroom. The viral theorists maintain that the kid would have caught cold if he had worn two mufflers and three pairs of wool socks inside his boots.

My own suspicion is that each of these theories, or rather a combination of them, is correct. There's little question that colds are viral infections and that the virus is transmitted through the air by victims who cough and sneeze or by contact with viruses lodged on hard surfaces. Yet, despite the lack of evidence that exposure causes colds, I'm inclined to side with the mothers and grandmothers who insist that children dress warmly when they go outdoors. This ambivalence arises partly because I think mothers and grandmothers know more about health than scientists and doctors and partly because it is an open question—in my mind—whether exposure lowers resistance to the viruses that are the direct cause of colds.

In any event, you have nothing to lose if you insist that your child dress appropriately in cold weather. You do have something to lose, though, if the doctor who correctly insists that your child's cold is viral proceeds to treat it with antibiotics, which are ineffective against viruses. I'll discuss that more fully later in this chapter.

SYMPTOMS OF COMMON COLD, INFLUENZA

The symptoms of the common cold, which vary in intensity from one child to another, are malaise, fatigue, runny nose, coughing and sneezing, bleary eyes, and usually a low-grade fever. Influenza, also viral in origin, is characterized by most of the same symptoms, plus vomiting, diarrhea, body aches, and high fever in many cases.

If the nasal secretions are clear, gray, or white, your child is probably the victim of a viral infection such as the common cold or influenza. If they are yellow or green, it indicates the presence of pus, which is indicative of bacterial sinusitis. Colds may also be complicated by other bacterial infections such as bronchitis and otitis media (middle ear infection).

Common colds and influenza do not require medical treatment, and the medications often used to treat them, as I have already suggested, will merely relieve symptoms. The effects of doing this may be counterproductive, because they interfere with the body's efforts to cure itself.

This is also true of viral pneumonia, sometimes known as "walking pneumonia," an ailment that neither you nor your doctor can identify except by X-ray. The symptoms are usually mild, and your child is in no danger from this form of pneumonia, except from the X-rays your doctor may order if you give him the opportunity. That is not the case, however, with bacterial pneumonia. This disease usually can be detected by fever above 102 and severe shortness of breath, followed by blueness of the skin. If your child develops these symptoms, there'll be no doubt in your mind that it is an emergency, and you should take him to a doctor or hospital emergency room at once.

Another respiratory ailment relatively common in children is croup. It is also viral in origin, and it can be identified by the metallic gasping sound that is heard when the child takes a breath; a hoarse, metallic cough; and an unusual pulling in of the chest on inspiration. If your child has croup, the symptoms will be relieved by taking him into the bathroom turning the shower on "hot," and allowing him to breathe the steamy air for 20 minutes. If that doesn't relieve the condition, suspect bacterial pneumonia and take him to the doctor.

Short of obviously severe respiratory difficulties, however, parents should avoid taking their child to the doctor or giving him over-the-counter medications for the treatment of symptoms. The drugs commonly used in the treatment of cold and influenza symptoms, whether prescribed by your doctor or purchased in the corner drugstore, fall into half a dozen classes. They include decongestants, expectorants, antihistamines, cough suppressants, pain relievers, and antibiotics. They have several things in common: they are unnecessary; they sometimes have undesirable or dangerous side effects; they may interfere with the body's own efforts to defeat the disease; and they are a waste of money. Frequently, several of the drugs are given in combination, even though one or more of them may address symptoms that your child doesn't have.

The decongestants, which are also known as *vasoconstrictors*, are prescribed to relieve difficulties with nasal breathing, which result from the swelling of the mucous membranes in the nasal passages. The decongestant opens the nasal passages by shrinking the swollen membranes. That gives temporary relief, but therein lies the problem. It is only temporary, and when the breathing difficulty recurs you are inclined to give your child more of the medication. Ultimately, there will be a rebound effect, and the congestion will be more severe than it was before you began the medication. A more sensible and risk-free approach to the relief of nasal congestion is the use of a humidifier or frequent visits to a steamy bathroom, as described earlier.

Antihistamines, often prescribed individually, or included in combination drugs, are used for the treatment of allergies. The body fights allergies by releasing natural histamine, which will produce watery eyes and a runny nose. Antihistamines stem the release of histamine, drying out the nasal membranes and hampering the body's effort to cure the cold. What the cold sufferer needs is more hydration, not less.

The expectorants are intended to liquefy mucus in the lungs so that it will be easier for your child to cough it up. Most of the preparations on the market that are alleged by their manufacturers to do this have yet to win approval from the Food and Drug Administration as being effective. It doesn't make much sense to buy a drug when the manufacturer can't prove that it works.

Several cold preparations contain the cough suppressant dextromethorphan hydrobromide, in amounts ranging from 3 mg to 20 mg. The FDA regards it as effective in suppressing coughs, but the question here is "Why would you want to?" Granted that the coughs may be annoying, the fact is that they serve a purpose. Why would you want to interfere with the body's mechanism for getting rid of the mucus that is congesting your child's lungs?

The principal pain relievers used in connection with colds and influenza are aspirin and acetaminophen. They are commonly given for two reasons: the reduction of fever, which I have already covered in detail; and the relief of the aches and pains often associated with influenza.

DANGER OF TREATING INFLUENZA WITH ASPIRIN

It's unlikely that you have ever heard this from your pediatrician, but the use of aspirin in connection with influenza is a risky business, indeed. This is also true of the antivomiting agents such as Compazine, Thorazine, and Tigan. Compazine and Thorazine are particularly dangerous drugs, originally developed for treating psychoses. They have been linked to Reye's syndrome, an often fatal disease of children. Its major manifestations are encephalitis and hepatitis. It is currently recommended that aspirin and these other drugs not be given during the flu season, much less to a child diagnosed as having influenza, because of their combined effect as a possible cause of Reye's syndrome.

I recommend against the use of any medication for the relief of symptoms associated with influenza and the common cold. If your child's discomfort becomes more than you can bear, use the appropriate medication for a day or two at most and limit the medications to those that are intended to relieve the symptom or symptoms that are troubling your child the most. Don't use the combination drugs that treat four or five symptoms at once.

Note also that many of the over-the-counter liquid cold remedies contain a high percentage of alcohol, and in some cases this may be the only ingredient that makes any sense. It may help the cold victim get some sleep, but even for children a shot of brandy will do it just as well, and the brandy won't be contaminated with a lot of drugs that your child doesn't need!

If you take your child to the pediatrician because he has influenza or the common cold, he is likely to prescribe drugs for the relief of one or more of the symptoms and probably a combination drug that addresses several symptoms at once. Many of the preparations that top the list of drugs most frequently prescribed are in this category, and in many cases their manufacturers are under orders from the FDA to prove that they are effective or take them off the market. Doctors continue to prescribe them, however, despite their dubious value and despite the fact that if all medication were avoided the patient would be better off.

Regrettably, that isn't the worst thing that can happen if you seek medical treatment when your child has a cold. There is a real danger that he will be given an antibiotic that is of no value in treating viral infections. Since the introduction of antibiotics a few decades ago, people the world over have come to regard them as the ultimate in life-saving drugs. At the outset they were used appropriately and, indeed, deserved the label *miracle drugs*. They conquered many of mankind's most feared infections, among them syphilis and gonorrhea, and some optimistic futurists foresaw the day when all infectious bacterial diseases would disappear from the face of the earth.

Alas, that was not to be. As is usually the case with doctors who are presented with a new form of treatment, the extreme soon became the mean, the antibiotics were prescribed for a broadening range of diseases, whether the drugs were effective in those applications or not. Several of them, originally developed for use in treating life-threatening bacterial diseases, are now prescribed for the treatment of colds and influenza.

Doctors could justifiably be condemned for prescribing antibiotics to treat viral diseases such as these if the only consequences were needless exposure to potentially dangerous side effects and the unnecessary expense. But these are the lesser consequences of what can only be described as medical idiocy. There are more threatening dual consequences of widespread, indiscriminate use of antibiotics: first, the development of antibiotic-resistant organisms in the community at large; second, if your child is needlessly and repeatedly exposed to antibiotics, he may ultimately be threatened by organisms that are resistant to all known forms of treatment.

WHY YOU SHOULD AVOID EXCESSIVE USE OF ANTIBIOTICS

Indiscriminate use of antibiotics by doctors, and particularly by pediatricians, is not at all uncommon. It may, in fact, be the rule rather than the exception. One hospital study of antibiotic usage found that they are given to one-third of all patients, and in 64 percent of the cases their use was not indicated or they were improperly administered in terms of drugs or dosage. The authors of the study observed that "A consequence of using large quantities of drugs capable of inhibiting the growth of microorganisms may be a selection of microbial flora resistant to these drugs. The appropriate use of such medication is of immediate importance to the patient and also of potential importance to patients who may be subjected to organisms resistant to available therapy. Antimicrobial drugs are unique in this regard, since their administration may thus affect their ultimate usefulness."

That's a complicated way of saying that antibiotics kill good germs as well as bad ones, permitting other bad ones that are resistant to antibiotics to take over and flourish. By improperly treating a disease that was treatable by other means the doctor produces a new disease that known antibiotics cannot control. That's a high price to pay for medical carelessness and incompetence.

Growing microbial resistance to antibiotics may ultimately set medical treatment back to the position it held before penicillin was introduced more than 40 years ago. In fact, the mortality rate for some infections such as septicemia (infection of the bloodstream) has already returned to the levels that prevailed before antibiotics came into use. Unless doctors change their behavior and become more rational and cautious in the use of antibiotics, we may see the day against which one Nobel prizewinning scientist warned. Professor Walter Gilbert, a Harvard chemist, said, "There may be a time down the road when 80 percent of infections will be resistant to all known antibiotics."

Why do so many doctors prescribe antibiotics for colds, influenza, and other viral conditions that these drugs won't cure? They tell each other that they do it because their patients want them to. That rationalization won't wash, however, because parents take their children to doctors to *get* medical advice, not to *give* it. A more likely probability is that doctors prescribe antibiotics for viral infections such as colds and influenza because nothing will cure them, but they've been taught always to give the patient *something*, lest their stature diminish in their patients' eyes. I can understand that, because I went through that medical school brainwashing myself. But I can't understand, if they still feel that compulsion, why they don't give their patient a placebo that would serve the same purpose and do no harm.

If you can't resist the temptation to take your cold afflicted child to the doctor, don't fail to defend him from antibiotics and other useless medications your doctor may prescribe. The odds are high that the doctor will prescribe them, because surveys have shown that as many as 95 percent of physicians give patients one or more prescriptions for the treatment of the common cold, and about 60 percent of the drugs are antibiotics. I say "defend him" because more is involved than simply paying for a useless medication. The incidence of side effects from antibiotics is far from low. One formal study revealed that vomiting, loose stools, and skin rash were experienced by 4 percent of children treated with penicillin G plus sulfisoxazole, and 29 percent of those receiving ampicillin. While most of the side effects were minor, severe reactions occurred in roughly 2 percent of the treated children. Percentages like that don't sound high to doctors, who are accustomed to prescribing some drugs that produce unwanted side effects in virtually everyone who takes them. However, they should sound high to parents who don't want to risk finding their children among the 2 percent who suffer severe reactions to drugs that don't do any good and shouldn't have been given in the first place.

Be particularly wary if your pediatrician prescribes tetracycline for your child. If your child is under eight years of age, and your doctor prescribes tetracycline for anything other than a life-threatening disease, leave his office at once. Find another pediatrician, because the one you have doesn't know what he is doing or doesn't care what he does.

In 1975 the American Academy of Pediatrics recommended against the use of tetracycline in children under the age of eight, because it can retard bone growth, damage the liver, and cause stomach upsets, nausea, diarrhea, vomiting, and skin rash. With extended use, it may also stain the child's teeth permanently yellow.

Always bear in mind, when considering whether to take your child to a doctor, or whether to use the drugs that he prescribes, that "what can be done will be done" by many doctors, whether it makes any sense or not. Many of the studies of antibiotic usage bear this out. One large city hospital used to require that the prescribing physician secure approval from the infectious disease consultant before antibiotics could be released from the pharmacy. When the restriction was removed the use of ampicillin increased eightfold. Similarly, when chloramphenicol was placed on a restricted list its use dropped by a factor of 10.

If I seem to have belabored the issue of antibiotic misuse, it is only because of its significance to the future health and well-being of your child. But I hope you will resist the use of other medications as well and quell the urge to give your pediatrician the chance to employ all of the worthless, opportunistic tricks he has in his bag. Where most respiratory illnesses are concerned, a pediatrician's training is a poor and potentially dangerous substitute for your own common sense.

DR. MENDELSOHN'S QUICK REFERENCE GUIDE TO COUGHS, COLDS, AND INFLUENZA

Common colds, influenza, and croup are caused by viruses and cannot be cured by any known medical treatment. They will usually respond to the body's own defense mechanisms within a few days and do not require medical attention. However, there are things you can do to relieve your child's discomfort and hasten his recovery when he is afflicted with one of these illnesses. Here are some suggestions for the management of colds and influenza.

1. Maintain a high level of humidity in the child's room or in your home. Be sure that the humidi-

fier is cleaned frequently, or it will spread irritants. If your child is troubled by difficulties with nasal breathing or a croupy cough, take him into the bathroom, close the door, turn the shower on—using the hottest setting—and allow him to breathe the steamy air for 20 minutes.

2. Make a determined effort to replace the fluids that your child loses from coughing, sneezing, and perspiring. Try to get him to drink eight ounces of fluid every hour. Fruit juices are best, because they have some nutritional value, but your objective is to get him to drink something, so give him anything he will tolerate—water, tea, or even soft drinks as a last resort, if he won't drink anything else.

3. Encourage your child to get plenty of rest. Try to keep him in bed during the early stages of his illness, but don't make a production of it. If he resists staying in bed, let him get up, but try to keep him from exerting himself too much. It won't even hurt to let him go outdoors, as long as he doesn't exercise too violently.

4. Avoid all medications, even though they may provide some mild relief of symptoms. If the child's misery becomes more than you can stand, give medications that are specific to the symptoms that trouble him most, not combination drugs that treat four or five symptoms. Don't give the medication for more than a day or two. Avoid cough drops, because they may produce side effects if taken excessively. They are apt to be, because to a child they taste like candy.

5. Try to remember, before you give in to the temptation to give some over-the-counter drug for the relief of symptoms, that you may be de-

feating your child's bodily efforts to cure himself. Most of what you can do with medications can be accomplished through constant attention to hydration and humidity.

6. Stay away from your doctor unless your child develops severe respiratory difficulties and blueness of the skin, which may indicate bacterial pneumonia. In that event, get him to a doctor or hospital emergency room at once.

7. Whether your child has a cold or not, try to make certain that he receives a balanced diet, rich in the nutrients and vitamins that he needs and as free as possible of the chemical additives that are present in most of the prepared foods sold today.

8. Remember that patience, loving attention, and tender reassurance will do more to make your sick child feel better than all the medicine on the pharmacy shelf!

11

The Mythical Menace of Strep Throat

It's an unusual child who lives in the north temperate zone and makes it through the winter without at least one sore throat. Scratchy, irritated throats can be painful and annoying—to parents, as well as to children. They often interfere with eating, talking, swallowing, and even sleeping, so they inevitably produce a succession of plaintive appeals for relief.

When your child is the victim, your instinctive response may well be to call your doctor. But if you yield to that impulse, you simply set the stage for medical intervention aimed at strep throat. Your doctor will almost certainly take a throat culture, and if it reveals the presence of strep, he'll probably prescribe an antibiotic. That may slightly shorten the course of the disease, but it will also increase the chances that your child will experience a succession of sore throats all winter long, for reasons I'll explain later.

Doctors aren't directly responsible for most sore throats, but they are responsible for the concern that parents feel when this symptom appears. The concern stems from the belief, inspired by doctors, that the soreness may be due to a streptococcal infection and that this condition, left untreated, may have grave consequences. These include acute nephritis or rheumatic fever and lifelong heart disease, both legitimate reasons for parental anxiety, so it is not surprising that parents reach for the telephone to call their doctor when a child's discomfort becomes acute.

As a parent, you need to know how you can relieve your fears without resorting needlessly to costly and potentially harmful professional help. You need facts that your doctor may neglect to provide about strep infections and sore throats.

First, you should be aware that sore throats, most of the time, are caused by viruses for which Modern Medicine has no cure. The only legitimate treatments a doctor can prescribe will not cure the sore throat. They will simply relieve the symptoms somewhat, and they are so simple and obvious that parents can perform them without any prior exposure to medical school.

Second, you should know that taking a culture to determine the presence of "strep" is a waste of your money and the doctor's time. It will *not* prove beyond doubt that your child has, or does not have, a strep infection. However, that question can be answered quite satisfactorily by clinical examination; an examination so simple that informed parents can conduct it themselves.

Third, the chances that your child will experience rheumatic fever, even if he has a strep infection, are extremely remote. During a quarter of a century in a pediatric practice that had more than 10,000 patient contacts a year, I saw only one case of rheumatic fever. In real life, the threat of rheumatic fever does not exist in most populations. The disease is rarely seen except among malnourished children living in the crowded conditions associated with desperate poverty.

Now, let's examine why I can confidently make these statements, which probably contradict most of what you have been told by your doctor, if, in fact, he's told you anything at all.

Because most sore throats are caused by viruses, they are not legitimately treatable by your doctor since no valid cure exists. They will respond to normal bodily defenses, however, and the symptoms usually disappear in three or four days.

A less frequent cause of sore throats is bacterial infection, almost invariably the streptococcus baccili. "Strep throat," as it is commonly known, will respond within 24–48 hours to treatment with penicillin. Without treatment, strep will surrender to antibiotics produced in the bloodstream and usually disappears in less than a week; antibiotics merely hasten the process a bit.

A third source of sore throats is three diseases that, when they are present, are a legitimate cause for parental concern. The first, relatively common compared to the others, is infectious mononucleosis. The second, diphtheria, was once a feared disease, but it has virtually disappeared. The third, leukemia, is relatively uncommon but is the most feared of all. All of these diseases demand attention by your physician, and you should see him promptly if the diagnostic instructions that follow lead you to suspect any of them. Mononucleosis and diphtheria are discussed fully in Chapter 19.

SORE THROAT CAUSES YOU CAN CONTROL

Finally, a surprising number of sore throats are caused by external conditions that you, as a parent, have considerable ability to control. These conditions produce irritation of the throat membranes, and soreness results. The principal offenders are dryness resulting from lack of humidity in the winter air; antihistamines you have administered to your child—with or without your doctor's advice—to relieve the symptoms of a cold; smoking or exposure to air filled with smoke; chemical pollution of the ambient air in the environment in which you live; and even too much screaming and yelling, which may irritate the vocal cords.

Sore throats caused by viruses are usually diagnosed by exclusion. If the symptoms associated with other causes are not present, and your doctor can't find another explanation for the condition, he attributes the ailment to a virus. In most cases that diagnosis will be correct.

No treatment is available that will cure a viral throat infection, and your doctor ought to tell you that. Some doctors, however, rather than admit they are helpless, may take a throat culture and begin an immediate course of penicillin treatment "because it may be strep throat."

The simplest way for you to forestall this possibility is to avoid your doctor unless there are clear indications that your child needs his help. Here's what you need to know to make that determination:

Characteristically, the onset of a viral infection is gradual, occurring over a period of one or two days. The first indication of an impending viral sore throat is usually a vague tingling sensation around the soft palate, which becomes evident upon swallowing. Within a day or two an annoying sore throat develops, often accompanied by a runny nose (usually a clear, watery fluid), mild fever, coughing, and swollen neck glands. If this is the sequence of events, you can reasonably assume that your child has a viral sore throat. Only if the symptoms persist for more than a week, or if respiratory difficulty emerges, is there any need to take your child to a doctor.

In contrast, bacterial infections emerge swiftly and within a few hours—rather than days—produce a high fever, swollen lymph glands in the area below the jaw, and extreme pain in the throat. They may not be accompanied by runny noses, coughs, and other common cold symptoms.

"STREP THROAT" NOT A SERIOUS CONDITION

Most cases of strep throat in children over age four can be diagnosed by looking for what doctors know as "the classic triad" of symptoms—pus on the tonsils and in the throat, swollen glands in the neck, and a temperature above 103. Pus is present when a normally pink throat appears to be fiery red, with spots of white or yellow that often look much like cottage cheese. If your child is less than four years old, you can't rely on a clinical examination to determine the presence of strep. A throat culture may determine it, but there is no point in taking one because, for reasons related to the immune response, children under four don't get rheumatic fever anyway.

If your child's sore throat symptoms persist for more than a week, which is beyond the normal course of the common viral and bacterial infections, take him to your doctor. This is simply a precaution to assure that he is not a victim of infectious mononucleosis or leukemia, which must be diagnosed by blood tests that you cannot perform. The delay in seeing your doctor will not increase the risk to your child, because in the early stages of a sore throat your doctor wouldn't and shouldn't perform these tests. That's because the treatment of mono is simply rest, which your sick child should be getting anyway, so early detection has no special value. Leukemia is so uncommon that indiscriminate testing for it is inappropriate, and the chances that your child has diphtheria are even more remote. If it is present, you will know it because the sore throat will evolve into severe respiratory difficulties, e.g., choking. Unless these symptoms appear, your doctor won't suspect diphtheria, either, because he probably has never seen a case.

Sore throats produced by environmental conditions will yield to the application of your own good common sense. If your child's sore throat is not accompanied by fever, glandular swelling, pus, or any other symptom, dry air is the first culprit you should suspect. During the winter, in northern climates, the humidity in the average home ranges around 15 percent. That number becomes more meaningful when you consider that the normal humidity in the Sahara desert is higher—18 percent! If dry air is your child's problem, spend your money on a good humidifier, not on office calls. You can exercise the same kind of judgment on the other environmental causes as well.

THROAT CULTURES, PENICILLIN, AND STREP THROAT

Parents, teachers, and other lay people have been educated by doctors to believe that, if a child with a strep infection is not treated, he is at grave risk of contracting rheumatic fever. This disease is a cause for concern primarily because it can produce rheumatic heart disease. When presented with a child who has a sore throat, the typical pediatrician will tell you, the parent, that he is going to take a throat culture to determine whether the child has "strep." He may also invoke the hazards of rheumatic fever as his rationale for doing so. What he won't tell you are all the reasons why taking a culture rarely makes sense.

He won't tell you, for example, that the sore throat is most likely to be caused by a virus and that taking a culture is a wasteful exercise if the classic triad is not present and there are no clinical indications of strep.

He won't tell you that, even if the culture is positive, it does not necessarily mean that your child has a strep infection. An average of 20 percent of perfectly healthy schoolchildren carry strep bacteria in their throats all winter long but do not develop the disease because of the natural immunity their systems have developed.

Your doctor probably won't tell you that under the best of circumstances only 85 percent of actual strep infections are identified by throat cultures and that when the lab work is done in the doctor's own office, rather than in a competent laboratory, the average accuracy may drop to as low as 50 percent. That's because those who perform lab work in doctor's offices are often relatively untrained and inexperienced and have only sporadic opportunities to run the tests.

Your doctor almost certainly won't tell you that, although the use of penicillin may shorten the course of the strep symptoms by three or four days, it may also cause recurrences of the infection all winter long. Antibiotics, while knocking out the strep bacilli, also prevent the development of the antibodies that are the body's natural defense against the disease. If the strep infection is not treated, but allowed to run its course, the body will produce antibodies to fight it that can continue to protect the child against reinfection during the remainder of the winter season. It is the penicillin's action against the antibodies that makes it effective in preventing rheumatic fever. The consequence of antibiotic treatment is that, if a child is subjected to a throat culture and penicillin at the beginning of the winter season, his tonsils will be the target of a cotton swab repeatedly, throughout the months to come. If one of your children has gone through a winter being treated for one sore throat after another, the treatment, rather than the bacilli, may be the real culprit.

Your doctor may ask you whether your child is allergic to penicillin; in fact, he's so fearful of malpractice suits that he almost certainly will. He probably won't tell you, however, about the potential consequences of an allergic reaction to the drug. Penicillin may produce diarrhea and rashes and, in rare instances, anaphylactic shock and death. If your child is receiving penicillin for the first time, be sure that your doctor is aware of this and that he monitors the child closely for any reaction that could lead to fatal shock. Remember, also, that while penicillin will not lose its effectiveness in the treatment of strep, indiscriminate and needless use of the drug may interfere with its efficiency in dealing with other, more dangerous bacteria later in your child's life. As I explained earlier, the patient may develop penicillin-resistant strains of bacteria, so that the drug won't work when it is really needed to save a life.

If your doctor gives you a prescription for oral penicillin, he may remember to warn you that it will be ineffective as a preventive of rheumatic fever unless the child takes it faithfully every four hours for 10 full days. However, the evidence is that, more often than not, this counsel goes unheeded, even if it is given. It is easy to understand why this is true. Typically, the antibiotic relieves the symptoms of a sore throat in a couple of days, as Mother Nature probably would have without the drug, and the parent often assumes that the medicine has done its job. It has, as far as the strep infection is concerned, but it won't be fully effective against the possibility of rheumatic fever unless it is taken for the full course prescribed.

Even knowing this, it is a remarkably determined parent who will continue to insist that the child take his medicine every four hours *for eight days* after he stopped feeling and acting sick. Repeated studies have shown that when penicillin is prescribed the compliance rates are well below 50 percent. That simply means that in more than half of the cases in which penicillin is given the patient doesn't continue taking it long enough for it to be effective against the disease—rheumatic fever, not strep—that it is supposed to prevent.

RHEUMATIC HEART DISEASE NO THREAT FOR MOST CHILDREN

If children were in significant danger of contracting rheumatic heart disease, noncompliance with the doctor's instructions would be a cause for concern. In real life it is a cause for concern only among the group at highest risk—the children in poverty-stricken households who are least likely to receive medical attention and, when they do, the least likely to take their medicine as long as they should.

However, despite overwhelming evidence that rheumatic fever has all but disappeared, except in the lower socioeconomic strata of society, doctors rarely tell their patients that it is a minimal risk. Parents are led, or at least allowed, to believe that rheumatic fever and the accompanying threat of lifelong heart disease is an imminent hazard for every child with a sore throat. That conclusion is contradicted by simple logic, as well as the statistical facts.

First of all, virtually all studies of the incidence of rheumatic fever among victims of strep throat have been done on closed populations in military bases and orphanages. It is well known that the epidemiology of closed populations is not typical of open ones. Yet these findings have been applied to the population at large, and millions have been treated for strep infections to prevent a disease that scarcely exists. It is fair to question whether the damage done by that treatment exceeds the risk that the penicillin is used to treat. Doctors are quick to warn parents of the dangers of rheumatic fever, but I don't know many who warn patients of the risks of the treatment they prescribe!

If rheumatic fever were a serious threat, one would assume that countless cases would emerge in a city as large and densely populated as New York, particularly since so many of its residents live in conditions of poverty. Such an assumption could hardly be further from the truth. In fact, only 57 rheumatic fever cases were seen at New York's famed Bellevue hospital between 1970 and 1977, and not a single case was identified in 1978, the most recent year for which I have data.

If pressed, doctors will acknowledge that the incidence of rheumatic heart disease is waning, but they are prone to attribute the decline to the availability of penicillin to prevent the disease. That assertion doesn't hold water, because the incidence of rheumatic fever began to drop long before penicillin came on the scene. Twenty-five years ago an attempt was made in the Chicago metropolitan area to establish a registry of rheumatic fever cases, and all doctors were asked to report those they treated. The effort was abandoned because no cases could be found in the affluent neighborhoods and suburbs of Chicago. The only cases reported were in the impoverished inner city, proving once again that it is only the children in poor families who are seriously at risk.

Studies have shown that the incidence of rheumatic fever is related to the density of children per room, which may also explain the results obtained in studies done in military installations and orphanages. Rheumatic fever is, indeed, a socioeconomic disease, and it is unlikely that the use of penicillin, even among the poor, will have much effect. The efficiency of penicillin varies with the nutritional state of the patient, and good nutrition is not a feature of poverty.

While it is clear that the incidence of cases diagnosed as rheumatic fever is diminishing, it is less certain whether this disease was ever a legitimate major threat. A study of cases diagnosed as rheumatic heart disease 40 years before revealed that 90 percent of the cases had been misdiagnosed because of misapplication of the classic criteria. Nine out of ten of the presumed victims of the disease didn't have it at all. Thus, it may be misleading to say that rheumatic heart disease is no longer a threat because, in fact, it never really was. This has significance for those who were diagnosed as having this disease many years ago and have been worrying about it ever since.

A final question for your doctor, if he still insists that rheumatic fever is a cause for concern: given the fact that as many as 15–50 percent of strep cases are not diagnosed and therefore not treated, and that half of those that are treated don't benefit because of the low compliance rate, where are all the people who should have contracted rheumatic fever because they had a strep throat?

THREE VIEWS OF THE TREATMENT OF STREP

A majority of doctors are divided into two camps on the appropriate treatment of strep throat. There is also a third camp, a lonely one, to which only a few of us belong.

One group of doctors insists that penicillin should be administered immediately in all cases of sore throat, without awaiting the results of the throat culture test. They note, correctly, that unless penicillin is given within 48–72 hours of the onset of symptoms it may not avert the possibility of rheumatic fever when it is finally used. Since the symptoms usually have been present for a period of time before the culture is taken, deferring the use of penicillin during the 24- to 48-hour wait for test results may render it ineffective.

The second group argues that penicillin should be withheld until the results of the throat culture are obtained. They point to the risks of penicillin, the hazards associated with its indiscriminate use, and the fact that patients shouldn't be told to waste their money on prescriptions they may not need.

The third camp, in which I place myself, holds that both throat cultures and antibiotics are to be avoided, because the hazards of treatment outweigh the remote possibility that your child will suffer any lasting effects even if he has a strep infection.

My position is simply the product of experience and observation over a quarter of a century. When I completed my medical education, I became associated with a pediatric practice that served a clientele along the affluent lakefront of Chicago. My senior partner was a learned and conscientious physician, Dr. Ralph Kunstadter. I was soon surprised to discover that he rarely took throat cultures, and when I asked him about it he said he considered them irrelevant and a waste of time.

Dr. Kunstadter had received his training 20 years earlier than I did, before the medical schools had totally abandoned Mother Nature, but I was imbued with everything I had learned about intervention. This led me to take throat cultures for a time, despite his example. I finally abandoned them, too, when I discovered that the results that I obtained after going to the trouble and putting my patients to the expense were no better than Dr. Kunstadter's. As I noted earlier, although we must have had 150,000 patient contacts during the 15 years we practiced together, only one case of rheumatic fever appeared. Obviously, risking damage to all the other children who had sore throats by treating them with penicillin, in order to prevent one case of rheumatic fever, would have been a poor trade-off.

WHY TONSILLECTOMIES SHOULD BE AVOIDED

Finally, a word about your child's tonsils—the interceptor of bacteria entering his throat, which may become infected as his body fights bacterial disease. Be on your guard if your child's doctor tries to persuade you that infection in his tonsils is an indication for their removal, for that is rarely the case.

For decades tonsillectomies were the bread-and-butter surgery of surgeons and pediatricians. During the 1930s doctors were doing between 1.5 million and 2 million tonsillectomies a year. Few children reached their teens with their tonsils intact, despite the fact that their removal could rarely be justified on legitimate medical grounds. For millions of children the consequences of this purposeless surgery were emotional trauma, loss of a natural defense against disease, and, in some cases, death.

The only absolute indications for tonsillectomy or for removal of the adenoids are malignancy or airway obstruction because the tonsils are so swollen that it becomes virtually impossible for your child to breathe. Yet, for many decades doctors performed them routinely, defending this irrational behavior with the unproven contention that failure to remove infected tonsils would subject the child to possible hearing loss or, at the very least, lead to recurrent sore throats.

The compulsion of pediatricians and surgeons to remove tonsils without justification was demonstrated in an experimental study conducted in the mid-40s. A group of pediatricians was asked to examine 1,000 children, and it was recommended that 611 of the kids have their tonsils removed. The remaining 389 were then taken to another group of pediatricians, who advised that 174 of them have their tonsils taken out. That left only 215 of the original 1,000, and a third group of pediatricians was asked to examine them. Although they had already been examined by two other doctors, tonsillectomies were recommended for 89 of them! If the charade had been continued for another round or two, surgery probably would have been recommended for the remaining 126 kids as well.

The tonsils and adenoids are lymphoid tissues, which are the primary site of the body's immunologic activity against disease. Because they are the interceptors of bacteria entering your child's throat, it is inevitable that they become infected, swollen, and inflamed. If they are removed, your child's first line of defense against infection is gone, and the responsibility is transferred to the lymph nodes in his neck. His body's immunologic competence is reduced and there may be an increased risk that your child will become a victim of Hodgkin's disease.

As a consequence of parental resistance resulting from media criticism of wanton removal of tonsils, the number of tonsillectomies now performed each year is only a third of what it used to be. Nevertheless, far too many are still being performed, and your child is a potential victim of one of them. I doubt that more than one child in 10,000 requires this surgery, yet hundreds of thousands of tonsillectomies are still performed every year. They result in 100–300 deaths, with a complication rate of 16 per 1,000 procedures.

I have long since concluded that locating the tonsils within easy reach of the surgeon's knife may have been God's only mistake! Unless your child's tonsils are so swollen that they interfere with his breathing, don't permit your doctor to perform a tonsillectomy unless he can offer convincing reasons for doing so. Even then I would recommend that you get a second opinion.

DR. MENDELSOHN'S QUICK REFERENCE GUIDE TO SORE THROATS

Sore throats, per se, although they may cause considerable discomfort, are not a serious condition, even if they are caused by a strep infection. They do not require medical treatment unless they persist in the presence of additional symptoms that may indicate a serious illness. Here is my advice to parents whose child develops a sore throat:

1. Don't rush your child to the doctor simply because he has a mild fever and a sore throat. See a doctor only if the symptoms persist for more than a week.

2. Replace the body fluids that are lost from perspiring, coughing, sneezing, nasal discharge, diarrhea, more rapid respiration, and loss of appetite. Give eight ounces of fluid every hour that the child is awake. That is a lot of fluid and perhaps more than he will want to take, so encourage him by offering a variety of options. The fluids can be nonfluoridated water, tea (ordinary or herbal), fruit and vegetable juices, soups, and even soft drinks as a last resort if that's all you can persuade him to swallow.

3. Maintain proper humidity in the child's room and, if possible, throughout the house. Humidifiers that supply cool steam vapor are excellent and safe. Remember, though, that it is important to keep the humidifier clean lest it begin circulating irritants that will further inflame the throat. You should try to raise the humidity in the child's room to at least 50 percent, although under some conditions that may be difficult.

4. If your child is complaining vociferously, you may want to do something to relieve his symptoms. The recommended dose of a simple analgesic agent such as Tylenol is appropriate. There are risks associated with this drug, but for temporary relief of pain I do not consider small quantities to be dangerous. An alternative that some mothers prefer, which often works as well, is a teaspoonful of liquor. For reasons that escape me, white liquors—gin and vodka— seem to be favored by those who make this substitution. Perhaps the parents don't want to waste their Jack Daniels on a kid!

5. My views on the suppression of fever have already been discussed, but let me remind you again that the fever associated with a disease is a mechanism the body employs to cure itself. It is unwise to interfere with it. Fevers below 105 do not pose a significant risk, other than that of convulsions. Convulsions are frightening but rarely dangerous and probably can't be avoided because they are not related to the height of fever but to the rate of ascent.

6. The penchant of doctors to prescribe aspirin or other drugs for the reduction of fever, which many of them do routinely, is one that I find appalling. Every doctor learns during the preclinical years of medical school that for every degree of rise in temperature the rate of travel of the disease-fighting leukocytes in the bloodstream is doubled. This process known as *leucotaxis*. I can't comprehend why a doctor would want to put the brakes on a mechanism that is striving to make his patient well.

7. Without treatment a sore throat—even if it is the result of a strep infection—should improve and disappear within a week or less. If it doesn't, see your doctor, because it may indicate the presence of a disease other than strep —infectious mononucleosis or, very rarely, diphtheria or leukemia.

   Mono is easily identified by blood tests, and the normal treatment is nothing more than good nutrition and bed rest. More severe cases may be treated with steroid hormones—usually prednisone—but this is radical and controversial treatment that should be used only in cases of extremely high risk. Diphtheria occurs so rarely that your doctor may not even suspect it, unless your child's ailment has reached the point of extreme respiratory difficulty. If your child experiences choking and is unable to breathe properly, rush him to the nearest hospital emergency room.

8. Doctors justify the use of penicillin to treat strep throat as a means of forestalling rheumatic heart disease. This condition is so rarely a consequence of strep infections that it does not warrant the treatment of the infection with antibiotics. However, if you do take your child to the doctor and he prescribes penicillin for treatment of a strep infection, the symptoms should begin to disappear within 24–48 hours. If they aren't gone in a week, inform your doctor. Your child's sore throat may be the result of a disease other than strep, and he should conduct the appropriate tests to determine whether this is the case.

9. Unless your child has chronic breathing difficulty because his throat is often obstructed by swollen tonsils, don't let your doctor perform a tonsillectomy without getting a second opinion indicating that one is really necessary. Your child's tonsils indicating that one is really necessary. Your child's tonsils are one of his body's natural defenses against disease, and he shouldn't part with them unless there is a clearly established need to do so.

12

Earaches:
Painful, Yes;
Dangerous, Rarely

Earaches can be the most painful of childhood illnesses. Your child may suffer greatly when he has one,
and because you feel so helpless and so fearful that the
infection may bring hearing loss or other consequences,
they can be agony for you, too.

Statistically otitis media (middle ear infection) is responsible for about 8 percent of all patient visits to pediatric practices and 17 percent of all infections that are
diagnosed. That does not mean, however, that 17 percent of all infections are otitis media, for it is probably
the most overdiagnosed and overtreated of all childhood
illnesses.

Most parents hasten to call the doctor when their
child complains of an earache. That's true even of parents who normally regard a call to the doctor as the last
resort when their child says he is sick. Their unusual
concern about earaches is prompted by the acute pain
that their child is suffering or the fear that it soon will
become acute. In addition, many parents hold the mistaken belief that ear infections may cause their children
to suffer the loss of hearing or develop mastoiditis, a
frightening relic of the medical past.

I am in no way critical of parents who hold these fears
because, for the most part, doctors reinforce them. Pedi-

atricians also, more often than not, diagnose ear infections where none exist. True, your child may experience a temporary hearing deficit as a result of recurrent ear infections during the winter months. But if he does, relax, because his full hearing will reappear long with the tulips in the spring. During more than 25 years in pediatric medicine I have never seen a case of permanent hearing loss as a result of ear infection. As for mastoiditis, which was a major concern of parents during my childhood years, I have yet to see a single case develop, whether the victims of the ear infection were treated or not. It has mysteriously disappeared.

In most cases ear pain is caused by pressure that develops when something—usually infection—interferes with the drainage of the ear through the eustachian tubes. Bacterial and viral infections can occur, however, in the ear canal (otitis externa), in the middle ear (otitis media), and in the inner ear. The inner ear infections rarely occur in children but in adults may involve vertigo, dizziness, and tinnitus (ear noises).

EARACHES CAUSED BY FOREIGN BODIES

Foreign bodies in the ear are another relatively common source of earches. They may cause pain themselves or lead to infection that causes pain. Small children seem to delight in shoving small objects into their ears and sometimes their nostrils. Someone even wrote a song about "beans in your ears." I can assure you that the offending objects are not limited to beans. Over the years I have invaded ear canals to remove pieces of paper, cotton balls, BB shot, vitamin pills, M & M candies, jelly beans, pieces of cereal, and even paper clips and safety pins.

If your child tells you he put something into his ear, or you have reason to suspect that he did, take him to your doctor at once. These foreign objects will rarely emerge by themselves, and it is dangerous for you to try to remove them. If you have no reason to suspect a foreign object, there is no need to seek medical treatment for the earache unless it has persisted for 48 hours or more.

Allergies are also a frequent component in the production of ear infection. They may predispose your child to bacterial infection. The most common culprit is cow's milk, in its natural form or as found in infant formula. It causes a swelling of the mucous membranes, which interferes with the drainage of secretions through the eustachian tube. Eventually infection results because of the accumulated secretions. Milk allergy is responsible for the high incidence of ear infections in bottlefed babies. However, allergies to other foods, dust, pollen, etc., can produce the same effects. So can allergy to chlorinated water in swimming pools.

Parents and doctors may also be responsible for injury to the ear canal and the eardrum because of their efforts to remove wax from the ear. This is rarely a necessary procedure, and when it is necessary, there are safe ways of doing it. If you want to avoid damaging your child's ear, I suggest you follow a simple rule that I have been giving to parents for years: "Never put anything into your child's ear that is smaller than your elbow!"

No one can provide a scientific explanation of why some children produce more ear wax than others, but they do. There are also racial differences in the quantity, consistency, and color of the wax found in ears. An accumulation of wax can sometimes cause mild, temporary hearing loss, but this rarely occurs in children.

The best way to remove ear wax is by inserting a few drops of hydrogen peroxide into the ear twice a day for two or three days. The child may complain about a bubbling or roaring sound when it is inserted, but it won't hurt him. Let the hydrogen peroxide remain in the ear for several minutes and then rinse the ear with gentle bursts of water from a syringe. You can also use a commercial preparation, Murine eardrops, but peroxide is less expensive and just as effective.

DANGERS OF REMOVING WAX FROM EARS

It is inadvisable for you or your doctor to use any kind of instrument to remove wax forcibly from your child's ears, even a cotton swab. Even though the package cautions them not to do it (in very small print), some parents are fond of using Q-Tips to remove wax from the ear canal. This is dangerous and unnecessary for several reasons:

1. You are going into a blind passage with a delicate membrane at the end, and you don't know how far to go.

2. The lining of the ear is a delicate structure with lots of glands and cilia that are there to keep the ear free of debris. The glands secrete mucous and oils. This lining is so sensitive that invading it, even with a soft cotton swab, is like driving a tank across your lawn.

3. The ear has its own mechanisms for moving noxious agents out of the ear canal. You interfere with these mechanisms when you attempt to clean the ear with a swab because you are likely to push wax and dirt back in and compact it so that the natural removal process is less effective. You may also cause physical damage to the ear canal or the eardrum itself.

Your pediatrician should also be discouraged from using an instrument to remove wax from your child's ears. He'll say he has to do it in order to see the eardrum and determine whether infection is present. That's not a valid reason, because one slip of his metal instrument, or one sudden head movement by a squirming child, could result in a punctured eardrum. Although this will heal itself, it may leave a scar, causing minor hearing loss.

Occasionally a child damages his eardrum by poking a sharp object, such as a pencil, into the ear canal. The eardrum virtually always heals itself without treatment. In all my years of practice I have never seen a case in which it didn't. Nevertheless, it is a wise precaution to see an ear specialist if this happens to your child. In extremely rare instances the damage may be sufficient to require surgical repair, but the doctor should be questioned closely before you accept surgical treatment, or even antibiotics, for an injury of this nature.

EARACHES CAUSED BY CHANGES IN PRESSURE

Another occasional source of earaches is the atmospheric pressure change that occurs when your child rides in airplanes or elevators. These pressure changes sometimes cause pain and temporary hearing loss, as you have undoubtedly observed on your own airplane flights. The symptoms disappear when internal and external pressure are equalized, but if they are not equalized, blockage of the eustachian tube can produce infection. Adults and older children can usually equalize the pressure by swallowing, yawning, chewing gum, or attempting to expel air from the nose while holding it firmly with the mouth closed. There is no evidence that this last procedure is harmful. Babies, who can't be instructed to follow any of these procedures, will usually avoid the symptoms if they are nursed during takeoff and landing. An alternative with infants is simply to give them something to chew or swallow.

HOW MOST DOCTORS
TREAT EARACHES

Let's turn now to what happens when your child has an earache and you take him to the doctor. When I was in medical school I was solemnly warned by my professors that untreated ear infections would result in deafness. For a long time, and just as solemnly, I transmitted this information to my patients and stuffed them with a succession of antibiotics, decongestants, and antihistamines. Later, when it began to become the vogue, I dutifully punctured the eardrums of my patients and inserted plastic tubes to facilitate drainage.

As the years passed I learned that many of my patients, perhaps the majority, failed to take their antibiotics for the time period prescribed, and many of them never got the prescription filled at all. In medical circles this kind of behavior is called "patient noncompliance," and it is frowned upon by doctors and pharmaceutical manufacturers alike. But what disturbed me more than noncompliance was the realization that my noncompliant patients recovered from their infections as rapidly as those who complied, and not one of them ever went deaf!

At first I consoled myself by invoking the standard line that all doctors are taught to recite when their patients get well by ignoring their advice: "You're lucky, that's all." Before long that rationalization no longer satisfied me, because so many untreated patients had recovered without medication that there couldn't be that much luck to go around.

That destroyed my faith in antibiotics, and I quit prescribing them, with no apparent negative effect on my patients. It wasn't long before I also lost my faith in tympanostomy—the plastic tubes. That happened because many mothers refused to let me insert them, and many others fell out shortly after I inserted them. In defiance of current medical opinion, those patients did just as well as those whose tubes remained in place for the prescribed period of time. My tympanostomy tubes joined the antibiotics on the shelf I reserve for drugs and procedures that are conceived for the benefit of doctors and drug manufacturers, not for patients.

Today I don't recommend antibiotics, decongestants, or antihistamines to any of my patients who have earaches. I actively oppose tympanostomies, and I teach my students to do the same. Their patients aren't losing their hearing because of ear infections, and neither are mine.

Unfortunately, we are among a minority of pediatricians, and the others are still going by the book. When your child has an earache, and you take him to the doctor, the pattern is usually set. After the nurse has taken your child's temperature the doctor will rush into the examining room, ask what the problem is, and then do a cursory physical examination. He'll check your child's throat, listen to his heart and lungs, and then peer through an otoscope to check the condition of his eardrums.

What he will see in the light shining from the end of the otoscope is the ear canal, which may or may not be inflamed, and the eardrum itself. If there is an infection beyond the ear canal, it will probably be in the middle ear. That's behind the eardrum, so the doctor won't be able to see the site of the actual infection, if there is any. He will make his diagnosis by observing the condition of the eardrum rather than the infected area itself.

Normally the eardrum is pearly white in color. When severe middle ear infection (otitis media) is present it will be a violent shade of red. When the doctor looks at your child's eardrum he may see one of these two colors or a range of shades of pink and red that lie in between. If he observes an eardrum that is beet red, he'll probably tell you that your child has a severe infection of the middle ear and give you a prescription for Amoxicillin, to be taken three times a day for 10 days. If he sees one of the lesser shades of pink or red, he'll probably diagnose it as a mild middle ear infection *and then proceed to treat it the same way.*

This doctor is treating your child improperly on two counts. First, the fact that an eardrum is pink or even mildly red does not mean that your child has a middle ear infection. The change in color can occur when a child is upset and crying, or because of fever due to a cause other than ear infection, or even because of an allergic reaction. A single observation of an eardrum that is slightly pink or red does not warrant diagnosing the problem of an ear infection, because the same eardrum may appear normally white if the doctor inspects it again an hour later.

The second mistake is treating the patient with antibiotics, whether his eardrum is pink, beet red, or even royal blue! The only case in which the use of antibiotics can remotely be justified is if the ear is actually discharging pus, which occurs in less than 1 percent of ear infections, and I'm not convinced that it can be justified even then.

A series of controlled studies have revealed that the use of antibiotics for treatment of ear infections makes no difference in terms of the important outcomes—hearing loss, spread of infection, or mastoiditis. Their use may slightly shorten the duration of pain and infection, but the trade-off is that the antibiotics also reduce the body's natural immune response. Consequently, in order to slightly reduce the duration of the infection, you increase the possibility that the child will have new infections every four to six weeks.

The most recent study I have seen reported cites the results of a double-blind experiment involving 171 children in the Netherlands. Half were treated with an antibiotic, and the other half were not. There was no significant difference in the clinical course of the disease —pain, temperature, discharge from the ear, or change in the appearance of the eardrum or hearing levels—between those treated without antibiotics and those who received them.

Some of my colleagues condemn me for the position I take on the use of antibiotics for treatment of ear infections. Sometimes they accuse me of endangering the lives of children by opposing their use. My response is, I believe, irrefutable. At least it has never been refuted. Here it is:

A majority of the ear infections experienced by children are not treated by doctors. Among those treated with antibiotics, the compliance rate is incredibly low. Children's Hospital, in Buffalo, New York, studied 300 children who were given prescriptions for antibiotics because of middle ear infections. Less than 50 percent actually received the amount that was prescribed. Only 22 of the 300 complied fully with the directions. In short, a majority of kids with ear infections aren't treated, and most of those who are treated with antibiotics don't follow directions so the antibiotics are ineffective. If antibiotics were really necessary to prevent hearing loss, hearing deficiencies would afflict most of the kids in the country.

I have discussed elsewhere the hazards of indiscriminate use of antibiotics. Those hazards prevail in the case of ear infections as well.

For years doctors have also prescribed oral decongestants and antihistamines in the treatment of ear infections. The principal drugs used are pseudoephedrine hydrochloride and chlorpheniramine maleate. The trade names of those most commonly prescribed are Actifed and Sudafed, and these drugs and others like them have been given to millions of children afflicted with ear infections or with the common cold. For years the Food and Drug Administration has questioned the value of these drugs and demanded that the manufacturers prove their worth or remove them from the market. Doctors keep right on prescribing them for children, nevertheless. In 1983, at the conclusion of a three-year study at the University of Pittsburgh, it was revealed that neither of these drugs was effective in the treatment of ear infections. More than 500 children were included in an experiment in which half were given these drugs and the other half a placebo. Both groups recovered at the same rate.

What I have tried to do in the preceding pages is reassure you that any fears you have had about the consequences of ear infections can be put aside and that the use of drugs in their treatment is not only unnecessary in most cases but may actually be counterproductive. The same advice goes for the surgical procedure already mentioned—tympanostomy—which today has become the surgery most commonly performed on children.

TYMPANOSTOMY RARELY IS JUSTIFIED

Pediatricians often use tympanostomy to treat chronic, recurrent middle ear infections where serious fluid is present. That's a clear fluid, not pus. Its purpose is to release the vacuum within the inner ear so that fluid will escape through the eustachian tubes. It's the same principle as punching a second opening in the top of a beer can so that the beer will flow freely out of the first one.

In doing the procedure, the doctor punctures a hole in the eardrum and inserts a polyethylene tube. The tube may be left in for weeks or even months. Sometimes it is removed deliberately; sometimes it falls out of its own accord. The principal justification for the procedure is the prevention of hearing loss, which is no justification at all.

Controlled studies have shown that when both ears are infected, and a tube is inserted in only one of them, the outcome for both ears is almost identical. Meanwhile the procedure itself carries many risks and side effects. Justified as a means of preventing hearing loss, tympanostomy can cause scarring and hardening of the eardrum, with resulting hearing loss. Incredibly, one of the side effects of this procedure, performed to cure recurrent otitis media, is *acute* otitis media!

WHAT TO DO IN THE MIDDLE OF THE NIGHT

What should you do when your child develops an earache and wakes you up in the middle of the night? First, don't seek medical attention immediately, even if he is experiencing severe pain. There is no worthwhile immediate treatment your doctor can provide that you can't provide yourself. Use a heating pad; insert two drops of heated (but not hot) olive oil in the child's ear every two hours; give whiskey by mouth, which will help the child sleep (Give 10 drops of whiskey to a small baby and up to one-half teaspoon to a larger one. The dose can be repeated in one hour and once more in another hour, if needed.); and, if severe pain continues, use the appropriate children's dose of acetaminophen. The object is to relieve the symptoms while the body defends itself.

If the pain persists after 48 hours, see your doctor to determine whether the cause of the pain might be a traumatic injury or the presence of a foreign body in the ear. If neither of these proves to be the cause of the earache, and no pus is draining from the ear, take your child home without further treatment and let nature take its course.

Most of my colleagues will regard this as a radical departure from accepted medical principles. I maintain —and I have given you the evidence that supports it— that it is the accepted medical principles that are radical and that my approach is conservative. Scientifically controlled studies have established that the conventional treatment of ear infections doesn't work and may damage the patient. While I can't provide any scientific evidence that olive oil and whiskey will cure ear infections, my patients will tell you that they do relieve pain, and I know that they won't do any harm.

Meanwhile, my colleagues' patients aren't losing their hearing because of ear infections, and neither are mine. But some of their patients are suffering hearing deficits as a direct result of the treatments they receive.

DR. MENDELSOHN'S QUICK
REFERENCE GUIDE TO EARACHES

Ear infections will not cause permanent hearing deficits, and mastoiditis is so rare a condition that most contemporary physicians have never seen a case.
Conventional treatment with antibiotics, other drugs,
and the surgical procedure known as tympanostomy is
no more effective than the body's own defenses in dealing with the disease. If your child complains of an earache, follow these procedures:

1. Wait 48 hours before you call your pediatrician.

2. Relieve the pain with a heating pad, two drops
   of heated olive oil (not hot) inserted in the ear
   canal, and the appropriate children's dose of acetaminophen if the pain becomes unbearable.
   Don't use aspirin because of the potential side
   effects. In 1955, as a young resident, I diagnosed my first case of aspirin intoxication. The
   child died, and I have been leery of aspirin ever
   since.

3. If the pain persists after 48 hours, see a doctor
   —not to treat infection, if that's what it proves
   to be, but to rule out the possibility of trauma or
   the presence of a foreign body.

4. Don't allow your doctor to use an instrument to
   remove wax from your child's ear and don't try
   to do it yourself.

5. If your doctor examines your child and finds a
   viral or bacterial infection, question the need for
   its use if he prescribes an antibiotic. If he finds a
   foreign body, let him remove it, but again question the need if he prescribes an antibiotic. If
   your child has a self-inflicted injury to the eardrum, your pediatrician may refer you to an ear

and throat specialist. Be suspicious and question the need if he recommends surgical treatment or antibiotics. In all my years of experience I have never seen a case in which either was necessary.

6. If your child has chronic, recurrent middle ear infection, it is probably because of allergies or the antibiotics he was previously given. If your doctor recommends tympanostomy, don't permit it without obtaining a second opinion. This procedure has replaced tonsillectomy as the favorite of pediatricians, but there is no reliable scientific evidence that it will do any good, and there's considerable evidence that it may cause further harm.

13

Protecting Your Child's Vision

Like most of us, you probably consider vision the most priceless of your senses and are appalled by the very thought that your child might lose his eyesight. That's an appropriate concern, so it is important for you to see he has proper eye care. It is also important that you know how to avoid improper treatment.

Vision is measured as a ratio of an individual eye's capacity related to what a normal eye should see. Thus, 20/20 vision means that an eye sees at 20 feet what it should see at that distance. If a child has 20/50 vision, he sees at 20 feet what he should be able to see from 50 feet away.

At birth, babies have some gross visual capacity, but their ability to distinguish details is limited. Their vision improves gradually until it reaches full capacity at about the age of five. A child's eyes are sufficiently developed to be capable of 20/20 vision at about six months, but the interaction between the eye and the brain is not yet developed well enough to provide vision of that quality. At the age of two a child's eyesight is about 20/70; at three, 20/30 or 20/40; at four, 20/25; it reaches 20/20 by the age of five, barring some visual problem.

Because some parents are concerned when they are told that their three-year-old has 20/40 vision, it is important for you to understand that it is not essential that anyone have 20/20 vision. Children can function quite well with 20/40 vision, and it is probable that the three-year-old with that level of visual capacity will have 20/20 vision at the age of five. It is also important to understand this because some doctors will prescribe corrective glasses for three-year-olds with 20/40 vision. That's unnecessary unless a specific eye defect requires correction or one eye sees better than the other so they don't focus properly. This should be corrected, or one eye may cease to function as it should.

The three common visual deficiences are nearsightedness (myopia), farsightedness (hyperopia), and astigmatism. All of these conditions are due to the shape of the eye and do not indicate either weakness or disease. If the distance between the cornea and the retina is too great, the eye focuses in front of the retina, not on it, causing nearsightedness. If the distance is too short, the eye focuses behind the retina, and the person is farsighted. Astigmatism is caused by an irregularity of the cornea or the lens. All of these conditions can be corrected with glasses or contact lenses, and none of them indicates a greater danger of eye disease in the future.

About 10 percent of children may need glasses for one or another of these conditions, but failure to wear corrective lenses will not cause the condition to worsen. Farsightedness often diminishes by the time a child becomes an adult at the age of 21; nearsightedness usually worsens but stabilizes at about the same age.

CROSS-EYES ARE USUALLY SELF-CORRECTING

During the first months of life a baby's eyes may function independently of each other, leading parents to fear that their child may be "cross-eyed" or "wall-eyed." This random movement is neither unusual nor abnormal, and by the third month of life the eyes should begin to function in unison when following moving objects around the room. Some children, however, display a condition known as *alternating strabismus*, in which one eye or the other sometimes wanders "out of synch." This condition is almost always self-correcting by the age of five, but if your child has it and you take him to the doctor, he may receive treatment, perhaps including surgery, that he doesn't need.

The condition can be serious if one of your child's eyes "sits in the corner" and is not functional at all. If this condition is not corrected, the function of that eye may be permanently impaired. This condition, known as *amblyopia*, is the absence of normal vision despite a normal eyeball and a normal optic nerve, because the eye does not transmit visual stimuli to the sensory portion of the brain that serves the eye. It can usually be averted by patching the good eye, which forces the use of the "lazy" one; through eye exercises (orthoptics); with glasses; and, in extreme cases—when all other measures fail—with surgery.

It is essential that true strabismus, which may lead to amblyopia, be corrected by the time your child reaches school age. If one of his eyes "sits in the corner," you should take him to a competent ophthalmologist for corrective measures. However, be certain that the doctor does not resort to surgery until all the less heroic measures have been tried and have failed.

Before you submit your child to treatment, however, be sure it is true strabismus you are dealing with, with one eye fixed in the corner, and not the relatively common alternating variety. Why? Because I have seen too many cases of alternating strabismus in two- and three-year-old children that doctors have insisted on correcting—even with surgery—despite the fact that the condition was almost certain to correct itself before the child reached the age of five.

Although the thrust of this book is to urge you to avoid unnecessary medical attention, I want to be equally firm in urging you to seek it when your child's condition demands it. Eye injuries are a case of this kind. When your child suffers a severe eye injury you should not attempt to treat it, and neither should your pediatrician. Take him at once to a competent ophthalmologist or a hospital emergency room that can summon one. Amateur treatment, whether by a parent or by a doctor who is not a specialist in the field, could result in permanent damage to the eye.

The only immediate treatment you should give for an eye injury is to apply a warm, moist compress and to bathe the eye with pure, sterile water in the case of chemical burns. Meanwhile, have someone phone the ophthalmologist or the hospital emergency room and describe the injury to determine whether there is anything further you should do before you leave for the hospital.

If you know the problem is simply a speck in the eye, and your child's tears don't remove it, try to wash it out. Pull back the lids and squirt boiled but cooled water (not *boiling* water) into the eye from a sterile eyedropper. Pay particular attention to the upper eyelid, because that is where foreign objects are most likely to lodge. If that doesn't work, try to keep your child from rubbing his eye until you can get him to the doctor. He could damage the eye if the offending object is sharp or abrasive.

MOST VISION PROBLEMS ARE OVERTREATED

Apart from actual eye injuries, doctors tend to overtreat other vision problems just as they do everything else. Many children suffer the nuisance of wearing glasses, and the ridicule of their playmates, because their doctors fit them with corrective lenses that they really don't need. One formal study of pediatric eye care involving 2,000 children and 300 pediatricians found that 7 out of 10 children with glasses did not actually benefit from them, presumably because their vision was not sufficiently impaired to require correction. An appalling 40 percent of those tested with their glasses on failed a visual acuity test!

Parents are put to substantial needless effort and expense by pediatricians who insist on routine eye examinations, sometimes demanding that they be given as often as once a year. The only beneficiary of this nonsense is the doctor who performs the examination. Your child, unless he is having obvious problems with his vision, does not need a routine eye examination, much less one every year.

It is a sensible precaution to have your child's eyes examined at about the age of 4, when testing becomes possible, and again at the age of 9 or 10. Beyond that, unless a vision problem is suspected at home or in school, no further examination should be necessary. For adults a conservative approach is to have a vision test every 10 years up to the age of 40 and every 5 years after that.

Doctors are also prone to overtreat eye illnesses, most of which are caused by allergies and irritation. The most common eye ailment in children is conjunctivitis, or "pinkeye," usually due to allergies, but sometimes to viral and bacterial infections as well. Children may also develop chronic red eyes because of exposure to tobacco smoke or other forms of air pollution, eyestrain, and inadequate sleep.

Allergic conjunctivitis may be caused by pollen, dust, animal danders, medications, cosmetics, food, chemical additives, and many other allergens. This type is usually characterized by itching and redness but not by a discharge from the eyes, other than tears. Another form of allergic conjunctivitis has its own self-explanatory name, "swimming pool conjunctivitis."

Vernal conjunctivitis, as the name implies, is seasonal. Typically, it appears in the spring, continues throughout the summer, and disappears during the winter months. The symptoms are itching, tearing, light sensitivity, and a mucous but not purulent discharge.

The final and most annoying category is catarrhal

conjunctivitis, which is contagious. The victim's eyes are red and sensitive to light; they itch and burn; and they discharge a thick mucus or pus that may collect on the edges of the eyelids. It is not unusual for children suffering from this form of conjunctivitis to awaken in the morning unable to open their eyes because the lids are cemented together. This can be a frightening condition for your children, so they need reassurance that their vision is not in danger. Obviously, because this condition is contagious, hygienic measures—such as not sharing towels—should be employed to avoid the spread of the disease to other members of the family.

There is no need for you to be able to distinguish between the types of conjunctivitis, but if your child is a frequent sufferer from this condition, you should suspect and look for an allergic cause. None of these conditions requires immediate medical attention, either, but if the purulent discharge of catarrhal conjunctivitis persists for several days, it may warrant a visit to the doctor for treatment with a topical antibiotic. In most cases your child's conjunctivitis will respond to gentle cleansing of the eyes with boiled (but *not* hot) water and a clean cloth.

If you suspect an allergic reaction, conduct a careful review of your child's history to try to identify the allergy that is responsible for the problem. Look for changes in activity, location, diet, medication, or other unusual conditions or events that preceded the onset of the problem. Once again, this is something that you can do more effectively than your doctor.

Styes, which are infections of the sebaceous glands at the edge of the eyelid, are another common affliction of children. At the outset a stye yields a sensation comparable to the presence of a foreign body in the eye. Subsequently there is tearing and a painful irritation and redness. Ultimately a pimplelike lesion appears at the edge of the eyelid. No medication is indicated, but the application of hot compresses for 10–15 minutes every few hours will usually localize the infection so that the stye drains and disappears. Boric acid or Epsom salts solutions are sometimes used, but plain boiled water will do just as well.

MYTHS ABOUT VISION

A lot of time and money is wasted because of myths about vision. Many of these beliefs are the source of needless friction between parents and children. Some people believe most of the following statements, and most people believe some of them, but there is no scientific evidence that any of them is true:

1. Reading in poor light will damage your eyes.

2. Too much reading will damage your eyes.

3. Sitting too close to a television screen will damage your eyes. (Avoid it anyway, because no objective research has been done on the long-term potential damage from low-level radiation.)

4. Reading in a moving vehicle will damage your eyes.

5. Exposure to flashbulbs and strong artificial light will damage your eyes.

6. Wearing another person's glasses will damage your eyes.

7. Wearing "dime store" glassess will damage your eyes.

8. Going without your glasses will damage your eyes.

9. Wearing glasses will progressively weaken your eyes.

10. If a foreign object isn't removed promptly, it may get lost behind your eye. (It can't, because the conjunctival membrane separates the visible part of the eye from the back of the socket. The only opening is the tiny lachrymal duct through which tears flow.)

11. Eating carrots will improve your vision. (If it helps you persuade your child to eat his vegetables, perpetuate the myth!)

So many situations arise in which parents must say, "Don't!" to their children that it is counterproductive to increase the friction by enforcing myths such as these.

DR. MENDELSOHN'S QUICK REFERENCE GUIDE TO EYE PROBLEMS

1. Unless you have a venereal disease, try to persuade your doctor not to place silver nitrate or antibiotic drops in your child's eyes at birth. (See pages 42–43) The benefits do not justify the risks.

2. If your child has no vision problems that become apparent at home or in school, there is no need for routine physical examinations at regular intervals. Schedule only two examinations during childhood—one at the age of four and the other at the age of nine.

3. If your newborn baby's eyes don't move in unison, don't be upset. The condition should correct itself by the third month of life. If the child continues to have alternating strabismus, in which one eye or the other sometimes moves randomly, do nothing. This condition is usually self-correcting by the age of four or five.

4. If your child's eye remains fixed in one corner, it can lead to amblyopia, a permanent visual disability, so see an ophthalmologist but resist surgery. Ask the doctor to try patching, orthoptics, and glasses first and resort to surgery only if all else fails.

5. If your child develops conjunctivitis, keep the eye clean by sponging it with sterile water on a clean cloth. Then try to identify an allergic cause for the condition. Stay away from your doctor unless there is a purulent discharge that persists for several days despite your efforts.

6. Treat styes with hot compresses to localize them so that the affected sebaceous gland will drain and heal. Medication is unnecessary.

14

Skin Problems:
The Curse of Adolescence

Skin ailments are rarely life-threatening, but they rank high in any catalog of parental concerns because of the emotional and psychological impact they often have on their victims—particularly adolescents. The disfiguring effects of acne, in particular, have made life miserable for millions of adolescents and adults, and this disease remains one of the most baffling conditions in pediatric medicine.

The first medical condition that troubles most new mothers is a skin problem—diaper rash. Stubborn cases, which make babies uncomfortable and irritable, can be extremely frustrating. Mothers, in despair, often respond by purchasing over-the-counter ointments or by consulting their pediatricians for treatment of this simple and common condition. Neither response is necessary, and both of them, in fact, may be harmful to the child.

It is symbolic of the practice of pediatric medicine that one of the first treatments an infant is likely to receive after he leaves the hospital is a classic example of pharmaceutical overkill. Virtually all doctors use some drugs needlessly; most doctors use some drugs recklessly; and the result is that dangerous overmedication has become the rule rather than the exception in American medical practice. Diaper rash is a simple condition that can and should be treated with simple measures, but

that concept is unacceptable to the pharmaceutical manufacturers and to many pediatricians as well. Present
them with a rosy, irritated backside and they'll unveil a
panoply of salves and ointments containing antibiotics,
cortisone, and hydrocortisone, with potential damaging
side effects that will *really* give you something to worry
about!

Prevention is the key to avoidance of diaper rash.
Don't use plastic or rubber pants or disposable diapers.
Use cloth diapers and be sure that they have been rinsed
free of any irritating detergents. Wash the baby carefully
with mild soap and water after each bowel movement
and expose his buttocks to the air as much as possible. If
a rash begins to develop despite these precautions, continue to follow the same procedures but dust his bottom
with ordinary cornstarch before rediapering. If that fails
to solve the problem, substitute zinc oxide ointment or
Lassar's paste, another zinc preparation, for the cornstarch. Finally, the obvious: monitor the condition of
your baby's diapers frequently, and if they are wet,
change them promptly.

If you observe these precautions faithfully, and the
diaper rash persists, there may be an underlying condition that requires medical treatment, but these cases are
unusual. An example is the rash caused by a yeast infection (often from antibiotic medications) for which treatment with a prescription ointment may be necessary.
Foods, such as cow's milk or soybean-based infant formulas, are frequently responsible. That's one of the almost countless arguments in favor of breastfeeding your
child. It greatly reduces the incidence of diaper rash and
other conditions stemming from dietary allergies.

Acne is at the other end of the spectrum of skin ailments that afflict children and adolescents. This disfiguring disease is the plague of countless teenagers and some
younger children and adults as well. The physical effects
are quite well understood, but the medical profession remains baffled by the underlying causes. Little or no
progress has been made in relieving the symptoms of

acne, much less curing it, without what are, to me, unacceptable risks.

WHY ACNE OCCURS

Acne is a disease of the sebaceous glands, which are located about ⅛ inch below the surface of the skin. Their function is to secrete an oily substance called *sebum*, which lubricates the hair and skin and inhibits the evaporation of water on the skin, which helps to stabilize body temperature. The composition of sebum is about half triglyceride, or ordinary fat. This is food for Corynebacterium acnes, a bacterium found in the hair follicles. The bacteria multiply, yielding by-products that produce irritation in the follicles. The process is complicated, but the result is that the pores become blocked, sebum accumulates, and the disease progresses from whiteheads to blackheads, to pustules, and ultimately—in about 2 percent of cases—to cysts. It is these cysts that produce heavy facial scarring, particularly if they are picked or squeezed, which triggers more infection.

There is a great deal of mythology about acne. Many people believe that blackheads are caused by an accumulation of dirt in the pores. They aren't; the black color is not caused by dirt but by an accumulation of the pigment melanin—the same substance that gives Caucasians a tan when they are exposed to sunlight. However, this belief leads many teenagers to scrub their faces until they are almost raw. Ordinary cleanliness *is* a virtue, but intense scrubbing with soap and water will not affect the course of acne, because it reaches only the surface of the skin and not the deeper area where the sebum is accumulating. Too much scrubbing may actually aggravate the condition.

Misconceptions about the role of diet are widespread among acne sufferers and even among doctors, for that matter. Some of the dietary beliefs may be useful, because they keep many kids from eating junk, but there is no scientific evidence that any category of food has a consistent effect in triggering or intensifying acne.

Over the years the finger has been pointed at chocolate, at fatty foods such as French fries, at peanuts, and at foods containing iodine. There is empirical evidence that some foods do aggravate the condition in some patients, but controlled studies do not point to any food allergy as a specific cause. Nevertheless, some individuals do appear to react to some foods, and when a specific trigger is identified as a possible cause it certainly should be avoided, despite what the research shows.

Some nutritionists are having modest success in the dietary management of acne, despite the lack of scientific evidence that it should work. Medical doctors may scoff at this, citing the studies that deny any dietary influence in the incidence of acne. Some even label it quackery. Meanwhile, they continue to treat their patients with their own forms of unscientific quackery, which won't stand up to the test of controlled studies, either.

MOST ACNE TREATMENTS ONLY MILDLY HELPFUL

More than 150 over-the-counter preparations are available for the treatment of acne. Most of the better-known ones contain benzoyl peroxide, which eliminates some of the oil and may offer mild relief to some patients. Even if it doesn't, your teenage son or daughter is better off using one of these preparations than some of the more hazardous but no more effective treatments that doctors prescribe. During the years that I have practiced I have watched doctors treat acne victims with antibiotics such as tetracycline and erythromycin; vitamin A in massive (and harmful) doses; zinc sulfate tablets; cortisone; injections of triamcinolone acetonide to drain the lesions; hormone therapy; ultraviolet light; lotions containing sulfur, sodium thiosulfate, salicylic acid in various combinations with alcohol; dermabrasion; chemical face peels; x-ray treatments; and even, incredibly, gynecological surgery! And after all of that witch-doctoring, some of them still have the nerve to call nutritionists quacks!

I won't get into the damage caused by all of these treatments, none of which really works, but let me illustrate what can happen to patients when doctors use unproven and untested treatments by discussing a few of them.

Twenty years ago tens of thousands of acne victims were given x-ray treatments in an effort to control or eliminate the disease. In fact, I prescribed these treatments myself. The results of this dangerous and irrational behavior are evident today in a virtual epidemic of thyroid tumors, some of them malignant, among those exposed to catastrophic radiation for this and other conditions.

Although they have abandoned x-ray therapy for acne, pediatricians and dermatologists have substituted other treatments that are largely ineffective and present hazards of their own. Various tetracycline preparations are being used, despite the risks. Prolonged use of this antibiotic may render your child's body susceptible to serious infection because its effects are not limited to harmful bacteria. It kills the protective bacteria in the body as well, opening the way to serious infections that were rarely seen 30–40 years ago. Tetracycline, when administered to young children, may also permanently yellow their teeth and even invade their bones.

Acne victims whose complexions are profusely pitted and scarred are also being urged to improve their appearance by dermabrasion. This procedure involves the use of sandpaper, wire brushes, and other abrasive material to remove a layer of skin containing the acne scars. The effectiveness of this procedure has never been established. A study reported in 1977 by a researcher at Houston's Baylor College of Medicine found that "Treatment of acne pitting and scarring by classic dermabrasion is, at best, somewhat disappointing; at worst it is unsuccessful and frequently accompanied by undesirable sequelae."

WHAT ABOUT ACCUTANE?

The newest actor on the acne treatment scene is a derivative of vitamin A, Cis-retinoic acid, which has been available in the United States by prescription since September 1982. It is marketed by the Swiss pharmaceutical firm, Hoffmann-LaRoche, under the trade name Accutane. It was estimated that doctors wrote 60,000 prescriptions for the drug during the first two months in which it was available.

Accutane differs from other drugs used in the treatment of acne in one major respect. *It works, but no one, including the manufacturer and the FDA, knows how or why.* In clinical trials it was effective in about 90 percent of the cases. That's the good news. The bad news is that it has such a frightening array of side effects that reputable dermatologists are extremely wary about using it. Too many others, however, are prescribing it with the same abandon that x-ray treatments were used 20 years ago, without fully apprising their patients of the potential consequences.

The risks and side effects are considerable. The *FDA drug bulletin* has pointed out that Accutane causes inflammation of the lips in more than 90 percent of the patients who use it. Up to 80 percent of the patients developed dryness of the skin or mucous membranes, 40 percent developed conjunctivitis, and almost 10 percent experienced a rash or thinning of the hair. Five percent experienced peeling of the palms of the hands and soles of the feet, skin infections, and increased susceptibility to sunburn.

My heart goes out to teenagers who are afflicted with acne and to sensitive and caring parents who must suffer the emotional and psychological consequences along with them. I can also understand why the teenage victim would gladly endure almost any risk to be able to look in the mirror and see a face that is blemish-free.

What you must consider, if it is your child who is affected, are the additional potential short- and long-term consequences of the drug. New ones emerge almost daily. If your teenager has acne, you must weigh the risks and benefits of Accutane and decide whether the benefits are worth the risks. In order to do that, however, you should be made aware of *all* the risks, not merely the obvious ones experienced by most of those who take the drug. It is doubtful that your child's doctor will give you this information in all of its troubling detail, so I will provide it here. My purpose is not to make your decision for you but to enable you to make an informed judgment about the use of this drug and decide whether you and your child are prepared to trade a short-term miracle for a potential long-term disaster.

The prescribing information on Accutane reveals not only that it acts on the skin but that high concentrations of the chemical reach many tissues other than those at which the treatment is directed. Experimental studies show that after seven days the presence of the drug can be detected in the liver, ureter, adrenal gland, ovaries, and lachrymal (tear) glands. The drug also produces reactions in the blood. Twenty-five percent of patients experienced an elevation in plasma triglycerides, 15 percent developed a decrease in high-density lipoproteins (HDL), and 7 percent showed an increase in cholesterol levels. These three factors are of major importance in the development of vascular disease of the heart and blood vessels. This side effect is of such concern that the manufacturer of Accutane recommends that "Blood lipid (fats) determinations should be performed before Accutane is given and then at weekly or biweekly intervals until the lipid response to Accutane is established."

Not only can Accutane affect the fatty elements in the bloodstream, but 40 percent of patients who received the drug showed evidence of other abnormal blood conditions which indicated that something was wrong without identifying precisely what the problem was. Thirteen percent developed high platelet counts, a change that can lead to disturbances in blood clotting. Ten to 20 percent showed decreases in red blood cell counts and white blood cell counts, the presence of white cells in the urine, and abnormal levels of blood enzymes (SGOT). Other users of Accutane (less than 10 percent) showed protein in the urine, red cells in the urine, or elevated blood sugars.

In clinical trials five patients treated with Accutane for more than two years showed skeletal abnormalities. Three adults had spine degeneration, and two children displayed X-ray findings of premature closure of the epiphyses. The last finding is of particular importance to adolescents, because the epiphysis is that part of the bone that normally stays open until full growth is achieved. Premature closing of the epiphysis will prevent a child from attaining normal stature. Another indicator of bone growth, the blood alkaline phosphatase level, is abnormal in 14 percent of Accutane-treated patients.

In 72 human patients who had normal pretreatment eye examinations, five developed corneal opacities (cataracts) while on Accutane.

Of potential importance to adolescent boys are experimental results in dogs showing degeneration of the testes after Accutane treatment, and also depression of sperm production. Studies evaluating the effects of Accutane on sperm production in humans are now being conducted.

POTENTIAL RISKS TO ADOLESCENT GIRLS

There is also potentially grave significance to adolescent girls and women in the propensity of the drug to cause fetal deformities in the offspring of experimental animals that receive it. In rabbits Accutane was toxic to the embryo and resulted in induced abortion. No adequate studies of Accutane have been done on pregnant women, but it is clear that the manufacturer is sensitive to the possibility that it could be another thalidomide. The prescribing information provided by the manufacturer cautions that "...patients who are pregnant or intend to become pregnant while undergoing treatment should not receive Accutane. Women of child-bearing potential should not be given Accutane unless an effective form of contraception is used, and they should be fully counseled on the potential risks to the fetus should they become pregnant while undergoing treatment. Should pregnancy occur during treatment, the physician and the patient should discuss the desirabilty of continuing the pregnancy." The manufacturer is concerned enough about fetal abnormalities to urge that "contraception be continued for one month or until a normal menstrual period has occurred following discontinuation of Accutane therapy."

There is no question that Accutane relieves or eliminates the symptoms of acne in most of those who use it, but the mechanism that produces this benefit, and causes the abundance of side effects, is unexplained. Because it has been in use for a relatively short time, the long-term consequences, of course, are not known. Looking at the myriad threats to your child that it poses, it is fair to note that its approval for human use is dubious, at best. If a chemical with as many dangerous properties as Accutane were sold as a treatment to remove wax from your kitchen floor, there would be a skull and crossbones on the label and a vivid warning, "Not to be taken internally." Yet doctors are apt to prescribe it with little or no warning at all.

This places an enormous responsibility on parents to guide their children in deciding whether to use the drug. A child with severe acne has an almost irresistible incentive to ignore the risks of Accutane. Furthermore, adolescents are more prone than adults to view disaster as something that happens only to others and choose the course of immediate self-gratification rather than that of common sense. Teenage automobile insurance rates, and adolescent use of street drugs, reflect those tendencies. Consequently, it is probably that a teenager with a badly marred face will discount the potential adverse consequences of using Accutane because of his compulsion to "get rid of the zits." He'll view the side effects as something that will be experienced by others and convince himself that "it won't happen to me." This makes it imperative that parents compel their child to consider thoroughly the risks of Accutane and participate with him in deciding whether the drug will be used.

My own behavior may be influenced somewhat by remorse over my ill-considered decision 30 years ago to prescribe X-ray treatment for acne, but I will not prescribe Accutane for my patients. The known risks are reason enough, and only the Lord knows the magnitude of the long-term damage that has yet to be disclosed.

EXPERIMENT WITH SAFE APPROACHES

The field of acne treatment is rich in theory and devoid of evidence of treatments that work, other than Accutane. Every doctor and health expert who treats acne has a catalog of treatments that he insists work for him. There is no scientific evidence that any of them do. Consequently, my strategy over the years has been to employ only the treatments that are least likely to damage the patient. Just like the more damaging ones, some of them work and some of them don't, but I don't know why, and neither does anyone else. Moreover, none of them requires medical supervision, so you can experiment until you find the most successful treatment without risks to your child and without any cost.

I noted earlier that there is no scientific evidence that the presence of acne is related to diet, yet in many individual cases nutritional approaches to the problem seem to work. Dr. Jonathan Wright, who writes an excellent column in *Prevention* magazine, offers one bit of evidence of a dietary relationship that, while not scientific, is convincing. He notes that acne was unknown among northern Canadian Eskimos until they shifted from a "primitive" to a civilized diet. At that point the incidence of acne among these Eskimos reached almost 100 percent. Dr. Wright is only one of many reputable physicians who believe that at the present low level of medical knowledge a nutritional approach is the only sensible way to deal with the disease.

"I have found only a few cases of acne (even bad ones)," Dr. Wright says, "which were resistant to treatment involving cleaning up the diet, avoiding food allergens, and adding such things as zinc, essential fatty acids, B-complex vitamins, and vitamin A. Even in many of the resistant cases, attention to factors of nutrient assimilation seems to help. In fact, I have hardly treated anyone in the last four or five years whose acne didn't settle down to a dull roar or to nothing at all with nutrition-related treatment."

I advise my patients who are victims of acne to pay particular attention to nutrition, not only to identify through elimination diets the foods that may aggravate the condition but to find a diet that will improve it. Don't bother talking to your doctor about nutrition, because he doesn't know anything about it and consequently doesn't believe in it. He believes in better living through chemistry and will probably prescribe tetracycline, hydrocortisone, or Accutane. Instead of seeing a doctor, read some good books on nutrition and try the procedures they recommend. Look for books by nutritionists Adele Davis, Carlton Fredericks, Michio Kushi, Paavo Airola, Dale Alexander, and Rudolph Ballentine.

Try diets that avoid refined sugar, white flour, and all processed foods containing chemical additives or preservatives of any kind. Carefully monitor your child's diet to determine whether his acne outbreaks coincide with the ingestion of any particular foods. Observe cleanliness but avoid excessive scrubbing of the affected areas, which may cause more harm than good. If you feel compelled to use some form of topical medication, see your druggist, not your doctor. The preparations that are sold over the counter probably won't do much good, but they are relatively safe compared to the medications a doctor or dermatologist may use.

OTHER SKIN CONDITIONS

I have devoted a lot of attention to acne because it is undoubtedly the single most troubling of childhood skin diseases, but there are a number of other common skin ailments that may one day concern you. One of the most innocuous of these is heat rash, which has no real medical consequences but upsets parents for cosmetic reasons. It can be so unsightly that it sends mothers to the pediatrician to get their beautiful babies back.

Heat rash is not a condition that requires the attention of a doctor; in fact, the less medical treatment it receives, the better. Heat rash in babies is usually the product of overdressing the child because of parental concern about "keeping the baby warm." Babies don't have to be kept any warmer than adults and will suffer no ill effects in normal room temperature if they wear nothing but a diaper or nothing at all.

If your baby develops heat rash, dress him lightly, or not at all, to give his skin maximum exposure to the air. Apply calamine lotion to sooth the itching. Use plain calamine lotion, not Caladryl, which contains an antihistamine in addition to the calamine lotion. Your child may be allergic to the antihistamine and suffer a variety of side effects, including the possibility of a skin rash to add to the one he already has. It is pointless to subject him to that possibility because there is no proof that the anithistamine will relieve itching any more effectively than the lotion used alone.

Another rather common skin disease, which usually develops in babies and very young children, is eczema. It appears as a rough, patchy, red rash; the skin becomes thick and scaly, and if it is scratched, a serum oozes from it that forms an unsightly crust. The conventional medical view is that eczema is hereditary, but I know of no scientific proof of that belief, and if it is correct, I believe it is an allergy that is inherited and not a tendency to eczema itself.

My own experience in treating eczema has demonstrated that the condition is of allergic origin and that it will usually clear up without treatment if the allergen or allergens that are causing it can be identified. In most cases the culprit is apt to be cow's milk or soybean-based formulas, but other foods and even other sources of allergy can be responsible. Breastfed babies rarely develop eczema.

Rather than use ointments or other medication if your child develops eczema, experiment with elimination diets to try to identify a food allergen that is causing the problem. Begin by withdrawing cow's milk and infant formula, and if the eczema disappears, eliminate them permanently from his diet. Even babies can survive quite nicely on meat-based formulas. If you are not breastfeeding your baby, any one of a number of books that are probably available at your local library will provide alternative diets that do not include milk or infant formulas.

STEROID HORMONE TREATMENT RISKY

If you take your child to the doctor because he has eczema, he is likely to give you a prescription for a topical steroid hormone, Kenalog, or for another steroid, prednisone. In stubborn cases, when all else fails, I have no objection to the use of Kenalog on small areas for a limited period of time—a few days at most. However, repeated and extended use on large areas of the skin may be dangerous because the steroid hormones in Kenalog are absorbed directly into the body through the skin.

Remember that both Kenalog and prednisone were developed to treat life-threatening conditions in which the benefits conceivably outweighed their severe potential side effects. In fact, the manufacturer's statement of the indications for the use of prednisone clearly states that its use should be restricted to "serious or life-threatening conditions...." The use of these drugs for treatment of eczema, acne, and even sunburn is another example of the pernicious tendency of American medicine to use extreme and dangerous measures to treat relatively innocuous conditions.

Impetigo is another childhood skin condition that is unsightly and annoying for children and their parents—the more so because it is of bacterial origin and contagious. It begins with a pimple that breaks and spreads, forming brown and yellowish scabs or crusts. The pimples usually appear on the face, making their presence even more annoying. Years ago doctors treated impetigo with gentian violet or potassium permanganate. It did nothing to cure the impetigo, but it covered up the infection by dyeing it purple, which was as ugly as the scabs. Today, doctors are apt to use antibiotics such as erythromycin and tetracycline, topically or systemically, to treat impetigo. There is no evidence that they are effective, either, but they are potentially harmful to your child for reasons that are explained elsewhere in this book.

Impetigo does not require medical treatment. Observe scrupulous cleanliness, to make sure that your child does not spread it to other members of the family, eliminate sugar from the diet, and wait for the condition to cure itself.

Hives are another condition of the skin, usually caused by allergies, that produce an itching sensation annoying to the victim. They appear in the form of welts, often all over the body, which may be white in the center because the swelling squeezes the blood out of the welt.

This affliction does not require medical attention; you can relieve the itching by applying calamine lotion to the welts or giving your child a cornstarch bath. The latter, although it is a folk remedy, not an accepted medical procedure, seems to work, but I don't know why. Then try to identify the allergy that is causing the problem, which you can do more effectively than your doctor. Allergens to suspect include medications, food, clothing, perfume and cosmetics, soap, chemical additives in food, and insect bites. If you take your child to a doctor for this ailment, he may prescribe cortisone or antihistamines, both of which are unnecessary and potentially harmful.

Fungal infections such as ringworm and athlete's foot may also appear in children as well as adults. Ringworm appears in circular patches of rough skin that are usually about the size of a nickel. When they are located on the scalp the hair within the circle may break off. Many doctors will treat this condition with antibiotics and antifungal agents such as griseofulvin. That's an improvement over the days when they treated it with x-rays that led to thyroid cancer, but it is still medical overkill. My advice: stay away from the doctor, observe scrupulous cleanliness, and let the condition get better by itself. That advice also applies to athlete's foot, but stubborn cases of this fungal infection can also be treated with over-the-counter preparations such as Desenex.

Because they are usually so active and spend so much time out of doors, children are more prone than adults to be exposed to poisonous plants and insect bites. They do not cause serious problems in most children, but in a few the allergic reaction may be severe and even potentially fatal.

If your child is exposed to poison ivy, poison, oak, or poison sumac, clusters of small blisters will appear on the areas of skin contacted by the poison, and a painful itching sensation results. This can be treated with calamine lotion and with frequent showers or cornstarch baths, in which a cup of two of cornstarch is added to a tub of water. If the exposed area is very extensive, and your child's reaction is severe, consult a doctor. He will probably treat the condition with topical or systemic cortisone or, if the reaction is dangerously severe, will hospitalize the child and give intravenous fluids. That's acceptable treatment if the condition is life-threatening, but cortisone should not be used for mild cases of poisoning because of the potential side effects and long-term consequences.

Stings and bites from bees, wasps, mosquitoes, and other insects produce a relatively mild, if painful, reaction in most victims. However, if your child is exceptionally allergic to bites of this kind, they can—although rarely—lead to death. The usual treatment is simply to wash the affected area with soap and water, apply calamine lotion, and use cold compresses to reduce the swelling. If the stinger is visible, it should be removed with a tweezer.

If your child has a severe reaction to insect bites, such as difficulty in breathing or a shocklike state, see a doctor. Also, try to limit his risk by staying away from areas in which he is likely to be exposed to insect bites. I have had patients whose reaction to insect bites was so severe that it produced generalized shock. I supplied the adolescents with adrenaline and a syringe that they could carry with them when they were required to enter high-risk areas, for use to avoid shock if they were bitten. Your doctor can do the same for you. In the case of younger children I gave kits to their parents.

Warts are perhaps the most mystifying—or even mystical—of disfiguring skin conditions. Many people still believe that they can be caused by handling toads (they can't), and old wives' tales abound about supernatural methods of removing them. What's mystical is the fact that almost any kind of supernatural treatment that the victim really believes in often seems to work. That may be pure coincidence, because warts usually disappear by themselves, without treatment, in time. However, the coincidences occur so frequently that one has to wonder whether the power of suggestion may not, indeed, be a cure.

Warts can be removed surgically, chemically, and with electrolysis, but no treatment is necessary for any but cosmetic reasons. They are caused by viruses and will usually stop growing and disappear if you give them time. If they are disabling, or intolerably disfiguring, see a dermatologist.

THE FACTS ABOUT SUNBURN

Finally, a word about sunburn, which in this nation of sun worshipers is probably the most common skin affliction of all. On any pleasant summer day millions of people can be found relaxing on the beach or at poolside, including a fair proportion who never go near the water. They're there to get a "healthy" tan, which they believe makes them more attractive. However, it's not all that healthy and over the long term won't make them attractive at all.

There are three negative consequences to overexposure to sunlight that should make you think twice about allowing your children to spend the summer baking in the sun. The first of these is a short-term consequence—painful sunburn—and the other two are long-term. One is the premature drying, wrinkling, hardening, and cracking effect of excess exposure to sunlight that will eventually make skin appear old before its time. The other is the possibility that excessive radiation, which is cumulative over time, will increase the possibility of cancer of the skin.

Sunlight contains two kinds of ultraviolet rays. One type is known as UVAs, which produce a tan, and the other as UVBs, which cause the skin to burn by breaking down the collagen and elastic fibers of the dermis, which is the underlying layer of skin. Initially, the only effect of the latter is a painful sunburn, but ultimately many people suffer premature aging effects, and some contract cancer of the skin.

Acute sunburn usually occurs during the first two days of a vacation among those who failed to limit their initial exposure and acquire a tan gradually by increasing their exposure on a daily basis. All it takes to ruin a Florida vacation is to permit your children to spend several hours in the sun on the first day or play at the pool or on the beach. The most dangerous hours are those between 10:00 A.M. and 2:00 P.M. and extremely hot days are the most risky because the effects of ultraviolet rays are increased by heat. Your child is more apt to get a severe sunburn if he is out in a boat, because of reflected rays. Suntan oils that do not contain a sunscreen that filters out the ultraviolet rays will not prevent sunburn and may even provoke it because the oil magnifies the sun's rays. Finally, don't assume that your child is safe on a cloudy day, because the clouds do not screen out all of the ultraviolet rays, even though they may filter them somewhat.

There are two ways to forestall the damaging effects of the sun's rays. The first, obviously, is to stay out of the sun or limit exposure to the periods of the year and the hours of the day when the sun's rays are less intense. The second is to protect your child's skin with a sunscreen that has an adequate Sun Protection Factor (SPF). These products should be labeled with an SPF number, which increases with the degree of protection offered. Some are as low as SPF 2, which offers very little protection; the most effective ones are SPF 15 or above. Pick one that matches the sensitivity of your child's skin.

Because the effects of the sun's radiation are cumulative, just as those from X-rays are, the risk of cancer increases with each exposure to the sun. In my view, however, your child's risk of developing cancer from exposure to sunlight is far less than his risk of developing it from X-rays, because sunlight does only surface damage and does not penetrate deeply into the body as X-rays do. Doctors typically tend to exaggerate the cancer hazards of sunshine, for which they can blame the patient, and minimize those of X-rays, for which they must take the blame. Be that as it may, the risk is there—from both causes—nonetheless. The link between skin cancer and exposure to sunlight is amply demonstrated by observation of the locations where most skin cancers occur. More than 90 percent are found on areas of the body such as the face, ears, backs of the hands, and back of the neck. People who spend a lot of time driving cars are most apt to get skin cancer on the left side of their faces, which are most exposed to the sun. Finally, if there is a history of skin cancer in your family, you are at greater risk.

How great is the risk that your child may ultimately get skin cancer if he spends too much time in the sun? Not great enough so you should lose any sleep over it. Because the lesions are visible, skin cancer is easily detected and diagnosed with a simple biopsy. The overwhelming majority of skin cancers are readily curable once they are detected. The case of melanoma, which can be dangerous because it may spread to other areas of the body, are relatively rare. They comprised only 2 percent of all the skin cancers diagnosed in the United States in 1982. You certainly don't want your child to develop skin cancer in later life, but the possibility that he might be seriously threatened by sunshine is not something that should worry you sick!

DR. MENDELSOHN'S QUICK REFERENCE GUIDE TO SKIN PROBLEMS

None of the common skin ailments experienced by children requires medical treatment. The exceptions are found in children with critical allergies to poisonous plants and insect bites, who may be subject to severe and even fatal shock. These children should receive medical attention at once. With this exception, the following common skin problems can be safely treated at home.

1. *Diaper rash:* Observe scrupulous cleanliness. Change diapers promptly when they are soiled or wet, dust the baby's skin with plain cornstarch, and expose the skin to the air as much as possible. In stubborn cases, apply zinc oxide ointment.

2. *Heat rash:* Dress the child loosely and lightly or not at all. Apply calamine lotion or bathe him in a tub of water containing one or two cups of cornstarch.

3. *Eczema:* Observe scrupulous cleanliness, avoid medications, and try to identify a diet-related cause. The condition will cure itself.

4. *Impetigo:* Observe scrupulous cleanliness. Take care to avoid spreading the infection to other members of the family. Eliminate sugar from the diet and wait for the condition to cure itself.

5. *Hives:* Relieve the itching with calamine lotion or cornstarch baths and try to identify a diet-related allergy or other allergy that is the cause.

6. *Insect bites:* Remove the stinger if it is visible and treat the site with calamine lotion to relieve the itching. If your child is severely allergic to insect bites, seek medical attention at once because of the danger of life-threatening shock. If your child has never been bitten before, monitor his reaction closely to determine whether he has a severe allergy to insect bites.

7. *Poison ivy, poison oak, etc.:* Wash the affected area with soap and water. Relieve itching with calamine lotion or cornstarch baths. If it is your

child's first exposure to poisonous plants, monitor his reaction and see a doctor at once if it is severe.

8. *Acne:* Closely review the history of your child's affliction to determine whether there is any cause-and-effect relationship between outbreaks of acne and food allergies or any similar cause. Experiment with elimination diets to determine whether food allergies may be the cause. Keep the lesions clean to minimize secondary infections, using mild, nonperfumed soap. Avoid excessive scrubbing and do not squeeze pimples. Unless you want to risk using Accutane, stay away from doctors, because they don't know any more about acne than you do and may prescribe risky, ineffective, expensive medications.

15

Skeletons in the Orthopedic Closet

Just as you are concerned about your child's intellectual and behavioral development, you are no doubt sensitive to every aspect of his physical appearance and development as well. You will observe with keen interest the age at which your baby first rolls over, stands up in his crib, crawls, and walks. If your child displays any unexpected physical characteristics, or lags in any area of motor skills, you may be concerned that something serious is wrong.

Don't mislead yourself by making developmental comparisons of your child with other children. If your neighbors' child is walking at an early age, and yours isn't, it doesn't mean that their offspring is smarter or physically superior to yours. The age span during which these developmental phenomena occur is quite broad, and variations rarely have any relationship to intellectual endowment or innate physical capacity.

Such comparisons are equally pointless when applied to the physiological structure of your child. First-time mothers, particularly, are apt to be almost clinical in the attention they pay to their child's physical appearance. They come to me expressing concern about their baby's flat feet, bowed legs, or "pigeon" toes, fearing that one or more of those conditions may be "abnormal" and require correction.

These presumed abnormalities create a bonanza for aggressive pediatricians and orthopedic specialists. Many doctors eagerly intervene with casts, braces, splints, corrective footwear, and even surgery, to "correct" conditions that would, in time correct themselves. If your child is the potential victim of this orthopedic overkill, protect him from it, because it is rarely necessary and may be psychologically traumatizing for the child who is labeled as needing this type of intervention.

The fact that your baby is bowlegged at the age of one does not mean that he'll resemble a "B movie" cowboy when he grows up!

Some of the fears that parents have about child development stem from myths that have been passed down in their families for generations. For example, there is a common belief that a child may develop bowed legs if he is encouraged to walk too soon. There is no scientific evidence that this is true. On the contrary, such encouragement probably will help the child develop a sense of balance at an earlier age. Equally false is the common belief that bulky diapers will cause a child's legs to become bowed. They won't, but they may keep the baby from having an accident in your lap!

At birth, virtually all babies have legs that are bowed and feet that toe in because of the fetal position that they assumed during the months before birth. Fat pads commonly present under their arches also give them the appearance of having flat feet. If parents are not familiar with the normal progression in the development of the lower limbs, it is not surprising that these seeming anomalies arouse concern.

DEVELOPMENT OF CHILD'S LEGS

After a baby escapes the confinement of his mother's womb his legs will pass through four stages of development. Up to the age of about one and one-half years there is a preponderance of bowed legs, which will begin to straighten out as the leg muscles are developed through walking and other physical activity. Between the ages of 1½ and 2 years there is usually a switch from bowed legs to knock-knees, and this knock-kneed appearance, persists between the ages of 2 and 12. Then, in adolescence, there is a balancing effect and the legs tend to straighten out.

Obviously, given this developmental progression, there are opportunities for doctors to intervene at any stage to treat conditions that will be self-correcting if the child is simply left alone. Doctors have a further advantage over patients because of the enormous variations in the development of one child and that of another. The development of the lower limbs falls into what one enlightened specialist has called "the borderland of orthopedics." There is no adequate definition of conditions that are normal and those that are abnormal, any more than there is a legitimate definition of "normal" for a child's nose or ears.

Unless your doctor can identify a specific physiological abnormality, and prove to your satisfaction that it requires treatment, no corrective measures for either bowed legs or knock-knees should be undertaken until your child enters his teens. In virtually all cases the condition will have corrected itself before that time.

If knock-knees do persist into adolescence, the most likely probability is that they have not straightened naturally because your child is overweight. In that event the kid doesn't need help from an orthopedist; he needs a dietician—a role that mothers are well equipped to assume. The exceptions are rare cases of clubfoot, neurogenic disease, or osteogenesis imperfecta, all of which present specific symptoms that go beyond presumed variations from the norm.

SHOES AREN'T IMPORTANT

The attention that many parents devote to the development of their children's feet is evident when you see a two-month-old baby lying in his crib wearing a $20 pair of high-topped shoes. The kid isn't going anywhere unaided, yet he is expensively equipped to run a four-minute mile! There's an element of vanity in this, of course, for baby shoes *are* cute. That's why so many of them wind up encased in bronze. But most parents do seem to believe that their children will have foot problems in later life if they aren't provided from birth with "proper shoes." Needless to say, the shoe manufacturers do nothing to discourage this conviction. The shoe industry benefits from the fact that a disproportionate share of the 600 million pairs of shoes sold in the United States each year are fitted to children and that a million or more are expensive, unnecessary corrective shoes.

Shoes, expensive or otherwise, are not essential to the proper development of the foot. Barefooted aborigines have better feet than millionaires shod by Gucci. Other than appearance, the only purpose shoes serve is to protect the feet from injury or the elements. Consequently, it is unnecessary and wasteful for you to invest in expensive shoes for your children for any reason other than appearance. A pair of inexpensive canvas sneakers will serve equally well. Expensive high-topped shoes will not help your child's feet develop properly, nor will inexpensive tennis shoes cause flat feet, fallen arches, or athlete's foot, as many parents seem to believe.

One survey of 104 normal infants brought to a clinic found that 87 percent were wearing shoes with high tops, 74 percent had shoes with hard soles, and 50 percent wore shoes with special arch supports. Seventy-three of the children wore shoes before they walked and 35 wore shoes before they could stand. None of the children derived any physical benefit from the shoes they wore. In fact, the high tops and stiff soles may have retarded the development of ankle strength and restricted their ability to learn to walk properly.

Wearing corrective shoes, in most cases, makes even less sense. There is no evidence that costly corrective footgear will correct any variation from normal, to the extent that "normal" can be defined. Except in the cases of clubfoot or other true deformities, corrective shoes provide no benefits to justify their cost. Meanwhile, a child who wears obviously corrective shoes that suggest a deformity may suffer emotional damage as a result. That goes for corrective casts and braces as well.

Although bowed legs, knock-knees, and pigeon toes are the most commonly treated orthopedic conditions in children, there are others that are grossly overtreated and often misdiagnosed. One of these, congenital hip dysplasia, occurs in infancy when the femur (thigh bone) is not correctly attached to the pelvis. Genuine hip dysplasia is most likely to occur in difficult breech deliveries, when the femur is dislocated from its socket. The condition should be corrected immediately by the obstetrician, who grasps the newborn child by its ankles so that the dislocated joint will snap back into place.

In most cases that is the end of the problem, if there was one. Congenital hip dysplasia, in which the dislocation persists, is quite uncommon, although it is frequently diagnosed. Studies indicate that it probably occurs in no more than one in 1,000 children and more likely in only one in 2,000. The condition is detected by placing the child on his back with his knees raised and his feet flat on the examining table. The knees are then pressed outward, and if one or both resist, dysplasia may be present. This can usually be corrected by placing a pillow or extra diapers as a form of splint between the baby's legs. Aggressive pediatricians however, may be reluctant to settle for this simple treatment. Many are prone to follow the problem with many repeat X-rays—exposing the child to imprudent radiation—and to utilize splints and casts to correct the problem. Beware of them, for this treatment is usually unnecessary, and the casts can cause muscle atrophy, circulatory disturbances, and emotional problems.

OVERDIAGNOSIS OF SCOLIOSIS

Another current fad among pediatricians is the diagnosis of scoliosis. The condition, found more often in girls than in boys, is a lateral (sideways) curvature of the spine. It can be detected visually by inspecting your child's posture from the rear to determine whether:

- one shoulder blade is higher than the other or one shoulder blade protrudes more than the other;

- the tilt of the child's waistline is abnormal, with a greater indentation on one side;

- the hips are tilted, with one more prominent than the other;

- there is an obvious curve to the spine;

- one side of the back or one shoulder is abnormally elevated when the child bends over.

In my early years of practice scoliosis was rarely diagnosed and even more rarely treated during the childhood years. Today the disease is fast becoming epidemic because doctors are ordering so many routine X-rays because mass screening has been introduced in some states. Doctors are diagnosing cases that never would have been picked up during an ordinary physical examination, and in many cases they are treating mild conditions for which no treatment is required.

I do not want to minimize the importance of treating scoliosis in cases that are severe. Left untreated, this condition in children may produce significant deformity in later life. However, I'm convinced that needless treatment of mild cases of scoliosis is probably a greater threat to children than failure to treat the cases that are severe.

If your child is diagnosed as having scoliosis, don't submit him to treatment without first making certain that treatment is justified by the degree of curvature that is present. Don't accept any form of treatment without studying the alternatives. In some cases it may be necessary to employ a "Milwaukee brace," an uncomfortable metal device that reaches from the chin to the hips and encircles the body, stretching and stabilizing the spine. I would not saddle a child with this contraption until all the less drastic measures had been explored. These include electronic biofeedback, exercises, deep muscle therapy, dance therapy, physiotherapy, and other less radical alternatives. Surgery, in my judgment, should be regarded as a last resort, employed only after all other methods of treatment have failed. Get a second opinion if surgery is recommended for your child.

My advice about the treatment of scoliosis echoes that which I give with respect to any ailment in which the parameters of normalcy and abnormality are relatively undefined. Many don't, but I believe doctors should observe the principle that "less is more." Don't take your doctor's recommendation of some draconian treatment at face value. Thoroughly explore the consequences of the treatment and the alternatives that are available and demand that your doctor defend the treatment he proposes to employ. Then, if you are still in doubt, a second opinion will be well worth the effort and the expense.

DR. MENDELSOHN'S QUICK REFERENCE GUIDE TO ORTHOPEDIC PROBLEMS

There are few adequate definitions of the characteristics that are "normal" or "abnormal" in the physical conformation of your child. Many seeming abnormalities of early childhood, such as bowed legs and pigeon toes, are merely stages in normal physical development. They rarely require medical attention and almost never require treatment of any kind. You'll avoid a lot of needless medical treatment and expense if you remember these things:

1. Infants almost always appear to have flat feet because they have a pad of fat beneath their arches. Even if their feet are truly flat, it is an inherited characteristic that does not require treatment or warrant the use of corrective shoes. Individuals with flat feet actually appear to have fewer foot problems than those whose arches are pronounced.

2. Virtually all babies are born with bowed legs, which straighten out naturally as the leg muscles develop. By the age of two, most children become knock-kneed, and this condition almost always corrects itself by the time the child reaches adolescence. Treatment for these conditions is not warranted unless they persist into the adolescent years.

3. Congenital hip dysplasia is extremely rare and seldom requires radical treatment with casts or surgery. Mild conditions are often overtreated. Don't permit your pediatrician to employ extreme measures without first assuring yourself that they are essential. In most cases no treatment is necessary, and in most others a simple pillow splint, or using extra diapers, will suffice.

4. Scoliosis is not serious unless the curvature of the spine is severe, but it is overtreated almost as often as it is overdiagnosed. If your child is diagnosed as a victim of scoliosis, don't accept surgical procedures or even bracing without first exploring all of the less radical treatment alternatives.

16

Accidental Injuries: *Medicine at Its Best*

It has always struck me as paradoxical that so many parents worry unduly about common, nonthreatening illnesses and yet give scant attention to the childhood accidents that kill more children than all the major children's diseases combined. More than 8,000 children under the age of 15 will die accidentally in the United States this year. Many of those accidents could be prevented, and many deaths avoided, if the proper measures were taken promptly after the accidents occurred.

At the end of this chapter you will find a list of guidelines that could help you save your child from accidental death or injury. Within the chapter itself you will find specific advice on how to deal with accidental emergencies, if your child has the misfortune to suffer one.

Most minor injuries do not require a doctor's attention, but emergency room treatment should be sought at once if your child's injury is severe. How do you tell the difference? The most important rule, if your child sustains an injury, is to avoid panic. That may not always be easy, because small cuts in some locations will bleed profusely, and it doesn't take much blood, spreading over a white T-shirt, to scare any parent half to death.

Nevertheless, you must try to remain calm, because your response to your child's trauma will require the exercise of immediate, sound judgment. You must decide whether the injury is severe enough to require medical treatment, whether to rush your child to the emergency room immediately or to call your doctor first, and whether to call an ambulance or take the child to the hospital in your car. Even in cases that are obviously so serious that they will require hospitalization, you need to decide whether any life-saving measures should be taken while you are awaiting the ambulance or before you put your child into the car.

On the following pages I will try to provide some guidelines that will help you determine the seriousness of injuries and the treatments you should use if a call or visit to the doctor is not needed. As in the case with all of the other advice given in this book, err on the side of caution when you are in doubt.

I urge emergency room treatment for serious injuries not only in order to get prompt treatment, but because I believe this is where you will find American medicine at its best. For the most part, emergency room doctors are better trained, more skilled, and more broadly experienced than other doctors. They are also accustomed to responding quickly to emergency situations. When he is in serious trouble, there is no better place to take your child.

CUTS AND ABRASIONS

Every parent knows that cut fingers and skinned knees are a common phenomenon among children, but I'm convinced that most parents don't know what to do about them. There is a common misconception that the use of antiseptics and even antibiotics is necessary to "prevent infection" when the skin is broken. Consequently, when a child cuts his finger or scrapes his knee, parents are inclined to rush to the medicine cabinet for some of the over-the-counter remedies that have been laid by for emergencies such as these. That's an ill-advised reaction because these home remedies are not necessary and may add insult to the injury and make it worse.

Most of the antiseptic preparations that are sold over the counter at your local drugstore—iodine, Mercurochrome, peroxide, and ointments of various compositions—may irritate body tissue but will have no significant effect on germs. The body has its own systems to fight infection, and they work quite effectively if you give them the chance.

What should you do when your child has a minor cut or scrape? Very little. Wash it gently with plain tap water to remove any dirt that may be present. Cover the wound with a clean bandage if that is necessary to stop the bleeding, but otherwise leave it exposed to the open air. No further treatment should be necessary for minor cuts and abrasions.

A doctor's services may be required, of course, if the wound is bleeding uncontrollably or is so severe that stitches may be required to facilitate healing or for cosmetic reasons. In that event your best bet is to head for a hospital emergency room.

Cases of severe bleeding constitute one type of emergency that you may have to handle quickly, without medical advice. If the blood is flowing from a vein, forget everything you have ever been told about applying tourniquets and try to stop the bleeding by applying pressure directly to the wound. Cover the affected area with a piece of clean cloth or gauze and apply pressure until the bleeding stops or until you can get the victim to the emergency room. Only when blood is spurting from an artery should you resort to the use of a tourniquet that totally cuts off the circulation to the limb. In those rare instances in which one must be used, it should be left in place for only a minute or two. If a tourniquet is left in place too long, it can result in loss of the affected limb.

Many parents wonder whether a tetanus inoculation is necessary every time their child suffers an abrasion or cut. Most children are inoculated against tetanus in early childhood (its the T in the DPT shot), but some doctors persist in giving tetanus booster shots when an injury occurs. In my youth I was told that tetanus was a threat if an injury occurred in a barnyard or from a rusty nail. Consequently, I gave tetanus booster shots whenever an injury of this nature was presented to me. I also gave booster shots, for preventive reasons, every 10 years.

Today I question whether booster shots are ever needed and even whether the administration of tetanus antitoxin makes any sense. There is no scientific evidence indicating how often tetanus boosters are required or whether they are required at all. Millions of American servicemen received tetanus inoculations when they entered service in World War II. Although four decades have passed, the evidence is that, with a few exceptions, their immunity has lasted until the present. That seems to be a powerful argument against the need for routine tetanus boosters at any scheduled interval shorter than 40 years!

BURNS

When I was a kid the standard home remedy for minor burns was the application of a coating of butter or lard. The theory was that this softened the affected skin and protected it from the air, which soothed the pain. A number of proprietary salves were also kept handy, which obviously had to be even better, because you could smell the medicine they contained. Today we recognize that there are several kinds of burns, categorized by the extent of the damage, and specific methods must be employed to deal with each of these categories.

When your child is burned the treatment you provide should have three objectives: the relief of pain, the prevention of infection, and avoidance or treatment of shock. It is important to know how to achieve these objectives in each of the three categories of burns.

First-degree burns affect only the outer layer of skin, which becomes red, sore, and tender but not blistered or charred. The immediate treatment is to immerse the affected area in cold water, which will lower the skin temperature and also help to relieve the pain. Subsequently a water-soluble antiseptic ointment or baking soda paste can be applied and covered with a gauze dressing. This is not medically necessary, but it will help relieve pain by reducing the exposure of the burn to air.

Second-degree burns are much more serious. They destroy the top layers of skin and damage some tissue as well. This can produce permanent scarring, and there is greater danger of infection because leakage of fluid from the blood causes the formation of blisters that can become infected when they break. A second-degree burn on a very small area, such as a child might receive from a cigarette, can be treated at home, but those involving larger areas of the body should receive prompt medical attention.

Third-degree burns are those in which there is charring and destruction of all of the layers of skin and even of some of the flesh beneath. The nerve endings are also sometimes destroyed so that there may be little or no pain. When second- and third-degree burns cover more than 10 percent of the skin area there is danger of death from shock or from subsequent infection.

Emergency treatment of second- and third-degree burns that cover large skin areas is difficult for parents to administer because of their reluctance to cause their child further pain. However, it is essential, and if your child is the victim, it is imperative that you steel yourself to do the things that should be done at once, before medical help arrives.

If professional medical attention cannot be obtained quickly, the best treatment is to immerse the burned area in cool (*not* ice cold) water as quick as you can. This serves two purposes. It will lower the temperature of the burned area so that thermal damage does not continue to progress, and it will provide some relief from pain by eliminating exposure to the air.

If it appears that the victim may go into shock, make

him remain in a prone position, keep him warm, and elevate his feet and legs unless there are associated head and chest injuries. *Do not* administer stimulants or liquids of any kind. The symptoms of shock for which you should be alert are a rapid pulse, facial pallor, cold, moist skin, trembling, and unusual thirst.

If the victim's clothing has adhered to the burned area, don't attempt to remove it. If blisters have formed, be careful not to break them, for that will multiply the risk of infection. Don't touch the burned area with your hands or any other object. Finally, don't apply lard, butter, ointments, antiseptics, or any other type of medication to the burned area. They will simply make it more difficult for the doctor to do his job.

Children are often afflicted with chemical burns when they become attracted to cleaning materials that are carelessly left within their reach. Many of these preparations contain strong acids, detergents, lye, and other harmful alkalies. If this happens to your child, the affected area should be flushed immediately with copious amounts of water. Be sure you immediately remove any clothing that may be saturated with the offending chemical. Then seek medical attention as a precautionary measure.

Another common source of severe burns to children is excessively hot tap water. There is no reason for the thermostat in a household hot water heater to be set above 125 degrees, but there is good evidence that most heaters are set above 130 degrees—a temperature that will produce severe skin burns in 30 seconds or less. Water heaters have been found in some households with the thermostats set at 160 degrees, a temperature that will cause a severe third-degree burn almost instantly.

Not infrequently, children left unattended in the bathtub turn on the hot water purposely or accidentally and then panic when they are engulfed in water that is painfully hot. If the thermostat of the hot water heater is set above 125 degrees, the results can be and often are fatal. It is estimated that more than 2,000 tap water scald burns require hospitalization every year and that as many as 15 percent of these burns prove to be fatal.

Why not check the thermostat on your water heater right now?

HEAD INJURIES

Head injuries sustained in falls, or when the head is struck accidentally by objects such as stones or baseball bats, are rarely serious. They seldom require medical treatment or X-rays, but close observation of the victim's reaction following the accident is required to make certain that no neurological damage has been done. Because they fear the possibility of lasting brain damage, many parents will rush their child to the doctor or hospital emergency room when he suffers an injury to the head. Children are often brought to me who have no observable symptoms, simply because they have fallen out of bed. These visits are seldom necessary and could be avoided if parents knew the symptoms to look for that justify medical attention for head injuries to a child.

If your child suffers a head injury, the first and most important question should be: Did he experience loss of consciousness, even briefly, following the injury? If he did, or if the accident occurred when he was alone and you don't know whether he did, take him to your doctor or hospital emergency room at once. An X-ray will probably be ordered to determine whether your child's skull was fractured in the accident. If the X-ray reveals a simple fracture, it is rarely serious, but if the fracture is depressed and pressing on the brain, further treatment or even surgery may be necessary.

If there was no period of unconsciousness, there is no need to call your doctor immediately. Many doctors routinely order X-rays when they are presented with a head injury, but this is not justified in the absence of symptoms other than the mere knowledge that there was an accident. Some doctors also order an electroencephalogram (EEG), despite the fact that the available evidence indicates that this is not of significant value in diagnosis.

It is important, though, following a head injury in which no loss of consciousness occurred, to observe your child carefully for at least 24 hours to determine whether there are other factors that indicate the need for medical attention. Look for symptoms by asking these questions:

- What is your child's level of consciousness? Is he alert or lethargic and difficult to arouse?

- Is there any abnormality in the size of his pupils? Is the pupil of one eye dilated more than the other and unresponsive when it is exposed to a bright light?

- Is your child experiencing double vision? (Do his eyes move in unison, as they should?)

- Can your child move all of his extremities in a normal manner?

- Is he having respiratory problems, indicated by unnatural breathing?

- Is there evidence of loss of coordination, dizziness, or difficulty maintaining balance?

- Is there any drainage of blood or clear fluid from your child's ears or nose?

- Is he experiencing a severe headache that does not diminish or increases in intensity?

If any of these symptoms are present, play it safe and see your doctor.

A final word to anxious mothers: don't assume it is a crisis if your child under five topples from a high chair or falls out of bed. Your child's screams are more apt to be from fright than from injury, for studies show that only 3 percent of the children who have this misfortune suffer injuries that warrant medical attention. Many of these were broken bones rather than injuries to the head. Be concerned about a head injury only if the child experiences a loss of consciousness.

POISONING

Ingestion of poison by children and deaths from poisoning have been reduced dramatically in the last quarter-century. This is due in part to the development of a network of poison control centers and to regulations requiring the use of childproof caps on many prescription and nonprescription drugs and household products. Despite this progress, however, more than 2 million cases of poisoning are reported in the United States every year, and a large percentage of them involve children. Most of them would not have occurred if the proper household precautions had been exercised.

At least three-fourths of the children who ingest poison will not require medical treatment if parents respond promptly and appropriately to the emergency. Your first step should be to try to identify the poisonous substance that was ingested and, if an antidote is specified on the label, administer it at once. Then call your local poison control center to determine whether anything further needs to be done.

If you identify the offending substance, but no antidote is suggested on the label, call your poison control center for instructions. If you have the container, keep it at hand, because you will probably be asked to read the label information. If you are told to take your child to a hospital emergency room take the container with you.

Home treatment, guided by experts in the poison control center, should be adequate in most cases. Most doctors are not expert in the treatment of poisoning cases. According to Dr. Richard Moriarity, director of the National Poison Center Network, "Most physicians have a very poor education [about poisoning] and very little training." Dr. Moriarity believes that about 85 percent of all poisoning cases are not life-threatening and could be handled at home.

The management of poisoning cases varies depending on the poison that was ingested, so it is important that advice be sought from a poison control center. If you have not already done so, look up the telephone number of your local center and add it to your list of emergency numbers. As a general rule, the objective in the treatment of poisoning cases is to remove as much of the poison from the system as possible and dilute or neutralize that which remains. In most cases this will require the use of a tablespoon of syrup of ipecac to induce vomiting, so it is wise to keep a supply on hand at all times. Don't administer it, however, until you have consulted the poison control center, because there are situations (as when corrosives have been swallowed) when vomiting is not recommended.

Vomiting should not be induced when the offending substance is a petroleum product, caustic, or strong acid. Petroleum products are likely to do more damage to the lungs than to the intestinal tract, so it is not advisable to bring them back up. As for caustics and acids, they burned your child's throat on the way down and you don't want to burn it further when they come back up.

Commonly ingested products for which vomiting should *not* be induced include gasoline, kerosene, naphtha, petroleum-based paint removers, turpentine, various polishers for furniture and automobiles, bug killers, drain and oven cleaners, ammonia and other bleaches, and products that contain sulfuric, nitric, hydrochloric, carbolic, and other strong acids. This list is not intended to be all-inclusive, so check with a poison control center before you induce vomiting to eliminate any poisonous substance.

What should you do if you discover your two-year-old with an empty medicine bottle in his hand? First, try to determine how many tablets or capsules the bottle may have contained. Then call the poison control center and give them the information you have. Don't assume, because the child exhibits no ill effects, that he is not in danger. The damage done by many drugs may not appear for several hours, and if you fail to act until the symptoms appear, you may be risking the life of your child.

The best way to protect your child is to keep him from being poisoned in the first place. This may involve some inconvenience in your household, but that is a small price to pay to assure that your child does not become a poisoning victim. Here are some suggestions that should be followed in every household where small children are present.

- Assume that all drugs and household products, however innocuous they may seem, are potentially dangerous if they are swallowed by an inquisitive child. Even children's vitamin tablets can be harmful if a child is tempted to eat a whole bottle of them.

- Put childproof catches on cabinets used for storing household products and lock up medicines and other dangerous substances. It is not enough to put them "out of reach."

- Don't leave dangerous substances unattended while you answer the telephone or the doorbell. Children have a way of getting into things, even if they have only a few seconds in which to do it.

- Keep medicines and household products in their original containers. This will prevent mistakes and assure that the label instructions are available in the event that the substance is accidentally ingested.

- Promptly dispose of empty containers and unused medications.

- When administering medications to your child, be sure the light is bright enough to read the label.

- When you have guests, be sure purses are placed where your child can't reach them. More than one child has been poisoned by medicine he found in a purse.

Occasionally a child is the victim of food poisoning that will make him very ill for a short time but has no serious consequences. The symptoms are vomiting, usually accompanied by diarrhea, that can't be explained by any prior evidence of an illness such as influenza. Unless there are obviously severe symptoms other than the two already mentioned, there is no need not seek medical attention or to treat your child with anything other than tender, loving care. You may relieve his thirst by allowing him to suck on ice chips, but don't give him anything to eat or drink for six hours after the vomiting has ceased. He may then have herbal teas, chicken broth, and boiled water, but withhold solid food until after he has had a good night's sleep. If the vomiting persists, and the child has lost more than 10 percent of his original weight, see a doctor. He may find it necessary to treat your child for dehydration.

SPRAINS, STRAINS, AND FRACTURES

The bone and muscle structure in children differs significantly from that of adults, and this affects the type of injury that occurs to arms and legs. Sprains, which involve the tearing or stretching of a ligament, are seldom seen in young children because the ligaments are not yet firmly attached to the bone. Growing children are more likely to suffer damage to the epiphysis, which is the soft end of the bone where growth occurs. If your child twists his wrist, knee, or ankle, and the swelling and pain persist for two days or more, see a doctor because, if it is a fracture of the epiphysis, it requires casting.

In children the outer layer of bone—called *perios-teum*—is relatively thick compared to that of adults, and also less brittle. Consequently, injuries that would produce a sharp break in adults, with the broken ends of the bone displaced, often result in "green-stick" fractures in children. The name is apt, because these breaks are comparable to the splintering that occurs when you break a green branch from a tree. Rather than snapping apart, the bone bends, producing many small longitudinal cracks at the point of fracture. This requires medical treatment.

If your child suffers a leg injury from twisting an ankle or a knee, there is no need to seek medical attention immediately. Delaying for a couple of days to see if the pain and swelling subside will not impede the treatment, if the injury proves to be a fracture and medical help must be sought. Encourage your child to keep his weight off the injured member and apply ice packs to the injured area to reduce the swelling. This will cease to be of value after an hour or so, and many doctors recommend that heat then be applied to improve the circulation in the injured member.

I should note, in all candor, that this is one of the many situations in which the "science" of medicine is less than precise. There is vast disagreement over whether the application of cold or the application of heat is the best treatment for a sprained ankle.

There is a classic story in medical circles about the doctor who told a patient to apply ice packs to his sprained ankle. The patient followed this advice for two days, with great inconvenience and discomfort, but the sprained ankle did not improve. He complained to his housekeeper about this lack of progress, and she advised him to apply heat to the ankle. The patient did, and the ankle began getting better almost immediately. The next time he saw his doctor, the following conversation ensued:

Patient: "Doctor, the last time I saw you you told me

to apply ice to my sprained ankle. I did, and it didn't do any good. Then my housekeeper told me to apply heat, and it worked right away."

Doctor: "Hmmm. That's funny. My housekeeper told me to use ice."

The point, of course, is that no one really knows which works best for sprained ankles—heat or cold. The important thing is to immobilize the ankle and wrap it with an elastic bandage to prevent motion that will aggravate the injury. Just be sure that the bandage is not applied so tightly that it cuts off circulation. Don't listen to anyone who tells you that the best treatment for a sprain is to have your child walk on it at once. Pain is nature's way of telling you that something is wrong, so if your child's ankle hurts, the message is "Keep off!"

If any injured member—ankle, knee, wrist, elbow, or shoulder—has not improved in a couple of days, see a doctor. The two-day wait will reduce the possibility that your child will undergo a needless X-ray yet assure that he does receive one if he really needs it. It is estimated that about 98 percent of the X-rays ordered for arm and leg injuries do not reveal a fracture, so it is obvious that many are ordered frivolously.

Parents whose children are receiving steroid treatment for asthma or other conditions should be alert to the possibility their child may suffer fractured ribs or vertebrae for no apparent reason. Extended use of steroids causes a reduction in bone density, and the asthmatic child who has been on steroid therapy for a year or more may actually suffer a rib fracture during a coughing bout. The National Asthma Center studied 128 children who had taken steroids for a year or more and found that 14 of them had suffered a total of 58 broken ribs or vertebrae. No fractures of this nature occurred among a control group of 54 other asthmatic children who had not received long-term steroid treatment.

If your child suffers a really serious injury in a fall from a tree or is hit by a car, and it appears that there may be a severe fracture or possible injury to his neck or spine, don't attempt to move him or pick him up. Cover him with a warm blanket to help avoid shock, and stem bleeding by applying pressure to the wound. Then make sure that an ambulance has been called, and await the arrival of trained paramedics who will know how to move your child safely and what emergency treatment should be given at the scene.

CHOKING

Infants and small children have a strong desire for oral gratification, which explains why they are so fond of popping small objects into their mouths. Sometimes these objects become lodged in their throats or are aspirated into their lungs, creating an emergency situation that demands action by anyone who is close at hand.

Cautious parents will avoid giving children toys that have small, removable parts; peanuts; or lozenge-type hard candies on which they might choke. However, you can't watch your kids every moment of the day so there is always the possibility, despite all your precautions, that a child will come upon something small enough to fit into his mouth. Sometimes the object gets stuck in his throat.

It is vital that you act promptly and properly when this occurs. The first step is to determine whether the child is able to talk and breathe. If he is, the airway is only partially obstructed. Rather than take any emergency measures that might jar the object into a more dangerous position, take the victim to a hospital emergency room and have it removed.

If the airway is totally obstructed so that the child cannot breathe, you don't have time to seek outside help. You must take emergency action yourself. First, inspect the child's throat to see if the obstacle is visible. If it is, and you think you can remove it with your fingers, try to do so, but don't try it if you think there is any risk that you will push it farther in.

If you can't reach the object, place the child over your lap or arm with his head and shoulders hanging down and slap him sharply between the shoulder blades with the heel of your hand. Do this three or four times to induce him to cough up the object. Remember, *never* slap an upright person on the back in an effort to remove an object, because it may force it farther into his airway or throat.

If this measure fails, try the Heimlich maneuver. Stand behind the child and put your arms around him, grasping your fists just below the center of his rib cage. Hold the thumb of one hand against his abdomen, and give a quick thrust inward and upward. The increase in air pressure in his lungs will often pop the object out of his throat.

Bear in mind that this maneuver was developed primarily for use with adults. If too much pressure is exerted on the abdomen of an infant or a small child, it can cause damage to internal organs—notably the liver. An alternative with infants is to place the child on his stomach in your lap and press sharply on his upper back to force air out of his lungs.

Many hospitals, and organizations such as the Red Cross, offer free instruction in cardiopulmonary resuscitation. Because of the frequency with which foreign objects are ingested by children, it would be prudent for you to enroll in a course if you have the opportunity.

ANIMAL BITES

If your child is bitten by a dog or any other animal, the wound should be washed immediately with soap and water and then held under running water for several minutes. Medical attention should then be sought as a precautionary measure or to close the wound with stitches, if that is required.

The most serious concern with animal bites is the possibility that the offending animal may have been infected with rabies. Make an immediate effort, if a dog was the culprit, to identify the animal and determine whether it has had rabies shots. If your child is bitten by a squirrel or some other wild animal, it is important to determine whether there is any evidence, in your area, that the offending species has been infected with rabies.

Rabies is caused by a filterable virus that has an affinity for nervous tissue so that it affects the spinal cord and the brain. The incubation period on humans can extend from 10 days to two years or more. The usual symptoms are uncontrollable excitement, fever, spasm in the muscles, larynx, and pharynx. As the disease progresses, the victim will salivate copiously and display unquenchable thirst but be unable to swallow water. That accounts for the term *hydrophobia*, a common lay term for the disease. Death often results from convulsions, exhaustion, or paralysis. Once the disease is present the only treatment is rest and sedation to forestall convulsions.

The choice to be made, if your child suffers an animal bite, is between the consequences of rabies and the consequences of the rabies shots that can be given to forestall the possibility that your child may become a victim of the disease. Because the disease is so horrible to contemplate, many parents accept rabies shots for their child even when there is no evidence that rabies was present in the animal that inflicted the bite.

If that decision is ever required of you, don't fail to consider the potential consequences of the shots. First, the side effects include extreme pain, which is not something you would wish on your child if it can be avoided. But of greater concern is the fact that rabies vaccine may produce fatal anaphylactic shock and severe paralysis that could incapacitate your child for life.

The possibility that the rabies vaccine will produce these dire consequences is remote, but so is the possibility that the victim of an animal bite will contract rabies, unless the offending animal is proven to be rabid. Tens of thousands of Americans are bitten by animals every year, but only a handful contract this dread disease.

Your choice is further complicated by the fact that, even if the offending animal is diagnosed as being rabid, there is a real possibility that the diagnosis may be invalid. A recent example of this occurred in Illinois, where the state department of public health incorrectly diagnosed rabies in 10 dogs and cats in the Chicago area. As a result, more than 100 persons submitted to painful and dangerous rabies shots, and many valuable dogs were needlessly destroyed. In some cases, the false diagnosis made by the state was confirmed by the federal Centers for Disease Control.

When a child is bitten by an unknown dog or by a wild animal, parents and physicians are presented with a frightening dilemma, one to which there is no "right" solution. During my years of pediatric practice I have passed through three stages in my response to the possiblity that the offending animal may be rabid. Today I give rabies shots only when the bite was inflicted by an animal known to be rabid; by a bat, a species likely to carry rabies; or by a wild animal of a species known to be rabid in the area in which the bite occurred.

So what are you, a parent, to do if your child is bitten by an animal? The only honest answer I can give, without playing God, is to tell you that it is a dilemma that you, with the help of your God, will have to resolve yourself. I can only tell you what I would do if one of my own beloved grandchildren were the victim: if the animal that inflicted the injury was rabid, or if there was a strong probability that it might have been, I would give the rabies vaccine. Unless those conditions prevailed, I would not.

Snakebites are also a threat in some areas of our country. When I was a child, boy scouts were taught to provide emergency treatment for snakebites by cutting an X in the wound and squeezing or sucking out the poison. I recall thinking that this was a gruesome act to contemplate. Today I know that there is no scientific evidence that this treatment will yield any benefits, nor is there any evidence that it will not. If the bite occurs in an isolated area where no medical help is available, nothing is lost by trying it. Otherwise, call your poison control center for instructions or rush your child to a doctor or hospital emergency room at once. It is important to try to identify the type of snake that bit your child and get him to a place where he can receive the appropriate anti-venin serum as quickly as possible.

FROSTBITE

Children seem to be less sensitive to cold than adults and, when they are enjoying themselves sledding or ski-ing, often stay out of doors longer than they should. Sometimes, when they come into the house, areas of the skin—particularly on their ears, nose, fingers, or toes—will appear totally white. When touched, this frostbitten area will be without feeling.

When I was a child there was a common belief that the proper treatment of frostbite was to rub the affected area with snow. That's one home remedy that makes ab-solutely no sense! The objective, when frostbite is present, is to warm the skin, not keep it cold. The ap-propriate treatment is to warm the injured member grad-ually by immersing it in water or soaking it with wet compresses that are at approximate body temperature. Hot water should not be used, because your purpose is to thaw the area gradually, and the frozen skin you are treating is not able to sense whether the water is too hot.

Cases of simple frostbite do not ordinarily require medical treatment, but extended overexposure to the cold, particularly when the victim fell asleep or became unconscious, usually requires treatment and hospitaliza-tion.

AUTOMOBILE ACCIDENTS

Although the types of injury that occur in automobile accidents have already been covered in this chapter, it would be inappropriate to end it without a word about auto safety. After the first few days of life, automobile accidents are the leading cause of death for children. Babies under one year of age are the most vulnerable, followed by children in the 1–6 year bracket, and then by those aged 6 to 12.

These statistics indicate why children are more vulnerable than adults in an auto accident. Because they weigh less, they are thrown about more by the force of the impact. This makes the use of the car seats for infants under 45 pounds, and safety belts for older children, a matter of critical importance. Don't make the mistake of believing that a baby is safe if you hold him in your lap. He should be in a car seat when you take him home from the hospital.

Approved car seats are now required by law in many states and should be in all of them. I say that as one who has had to try to mend the appalling injuries that result from auto accidents. All of us are inclined to think that accidents are something that happens to others. Yet in 1981 auto accidents caused 1,900,000 disabling injuries, 1,750,000 temporary total disabilities, 150,000 permanent impairments, and 50,800 fatalities. With a staggering incidence of death, injury, and disability such as that, it's apparent that an auto accident might happen to any of us, or to our children.

DR. MENDELSOHN'S QUICK
REFERENCE GUIDE TO
ACCIDENTAL INJURES

The vast majority of accidental injuries do not require medical attention if parents are familiar with the treatment they can apply at home. However, judgment must be exercised to determine which injuries are extensive and serious enough to demand medical care. Study the information provided in each of the headings in this chapter, and you will be able to apply the appropriate treatment and exercise the considered judgment that will be required if an accident befalls your child.

HOUSEHOLD SAFETY PRECAUTIONS

- Teach your children the fundamentals of safety and set a good example for them yourself.

- Don't leave babies and young children unsupervised.

- Check the thermostat on your water heater and make certain it is not set above 125 degrees.

- Do not allow allow children to play with matches or use the stove without permission. Make certain that the handles on cooking pans are not where children can reach them. Keep hot fluids out of the reach of children.

- Keep scissors and knives where small children can't reach them.

- Keep power tools and sharp hand tools where children cannot reach them.

- Unload all firearms, lock them up, and lock up the ammunition in a separate location.

- Cover electrical outlets and don't keep electrical appliances in the bathroom.

- Check all toys to be sure they don't present hazards.

- Keep all medicines in locked cabinets and store household cleaning products in cabinets that are locked or have childproof latches.

- Make certain that window screen and porch railings are secure.

- Don't leave toys on the staircase or use loose rugs on or near stairways.

- Keep the sides up when your baby is in the crib, strap him into his high chair, and place gates at the top and bottom of each stairway when he begins to crawl.

- Fill holes that appear in your yard and repair broken sidewalks immediately.

- If you have a pool, don't permit your children to swim unattended, be sure it is securely fenced, and don't allow your children or their guests to run on the slippery deck.

- Post a list of emergency numbers next to each of your telephones. It should include the telephone numbers of your pediatrician, the local ambulance service, the hospital emergency room, the poison control center, and the fire and police departments. This could save valuable time when an accident occurs.

- When traveling in an automobile, make sure that your child under 45 pounds is strapped into an approved car seat and that every member of your family has his or her seat belt securely fastened.

17

Asthma and Allergies: *Try Diet, Not Drugs*

You won't find the word *allergy* in Shakespeare or even in the English literature of a century ago. The medical concept that allergies are responsible for many human ailments is a relatively new one. Yet it is not new enough to excuse the failure of most doctors to accord it an appropriate role in differential diagnosis. It is a sad fact that allergies and nutrition—two major forces in human health—receive little attention in medical school and constitute an area of vast ignorance in contemporary medical practice.

Although we often are not aware of it, most of us are allergic to things in the food we eat and the air we breathe. Because of medical ignorance, however, many diseases that could be managed by identifying and avoiding the allergens that cause them are treated, instead, with dangerous drugs and even surgery. In many cases this unnecessary treatment is worse than the disease being treated.

The most common allergies are those that produce stuffed-up, runny noses, sneezing, and coughing. When these symptoms appear only in the fall of the year we assume that the culprit is pollen in the air and call the ailment *hay fever*. However, some people suffer from these symptoms throughout the year, with chronic nasal obstructions that may lead to other infections (sinus, etc.) as well. In those cases allergens other than pollen are obviously responsible.

Some allergens are found in the environment in which we live and others in the food we eat. The environmental allergies include pollen and molds; air pollution from heating fuel, automobile exhausts, and tobacco smoke; animal dander (minute scales from hair, feathers, or skin); household dust; drinking water (chlorine); fabrics in clothing, blankets, quilts (particularly wool); cosmetics and soaps; chemical sprays; and insect bites, to name some of the most common offenders.

Food allergies cover a broad range, with cow's milk at the top of the list. Other foods that produce allergic reactions in some children include corn products, wheat fractions, gluten, eggs, fish, tomatoes, garlic, citrus fruits, and the chemical additives, preservatives, stabilizers, coloring, and flavoring that are found in most processed foods.

ALLERGIES PRODUCE MANY SYMPTOMS IN CHILDREN

Children are particularly susceptible to allergic reactions that may produce such diverse symptoms as headache, migraine, eye pain and blurred vision, vertigo, hearing loss, tachycardia (rapid heartbeat), nausea, vomiting, heartburn, diarrhea, abdominal pain, allergic cystitis (blood in urine), fatigue, muscle weakness, bed-wetting, learning disorders, insomnia, hyperactivity, and poor memory. Bottlefed babies are at least 20 times as susceptible to allergies as children who are breastfed.

All doctors will assume that allergies are responsible for diseases such as asthma and hay fever, and most will suspect allergies as the cause of some skin conditions, but many fail to consider the possibility of allergies when your child has the other symptoms cited above. Instead, they shoot at the wrong target and give him drugs for the relief of symptoms rather than doing the medical detective work that might have identified a food or environmental allergy as the culprit that was making your child sick.

While failure to consider allergies as the potential cause of illness can lead to false diagnosis and inappropriate treatment, recognition of the possibility may be equally dangerous. A pediatrician's suspicion of allergy usually leads him to refer your child to an allergist whose response may also be inappropriate. Many allergists abuse skin testing by haphazardly performing dozens of uncomfortable, costly, and potentially dangerous skin tests. These tests, especially for food allergies, are notoriously inaccurate and totally inappropriate when given—as they often are—for potential allergens to which your child is not even exposed. They have legitimacy and value in confirming suspected allergies that have been identified by other means, but indiscriminate testing is not to be condoned.

Testing, however, is only part of the problem. The treatments that follow may be worse than the symptoms they are supposed to relieve. If scratch tests reveal that your child is allergic to household dust, it obviously makes sense to provide him with the most dust-free environment that can be contrived. Elimination of suspect foods also makes sense if it is carried out as part of an elimination diet to validate or invalidate the tests. However, it is pointless to eliminate nutritious foods permanently without testing your child's reaction to them to confirm the validity of the tests. That being the case, why give the tests? Why not use an elimination diet to determine your child's reaction to specific foods and skip the scratch tests?

The real hazard, when you take your child to an allergist, is the probability that he will prescribe desensitization shots or treatment with drugs such as antihistamines, adrenal corticosteroid hormones such as cortisone or prednisone, or xanthine derivatives such as theophylline.

The value of administering allergy desensitization

shots is extremely controversial, and the long-term consequences are unknown. The few controlled studies that have been made of their effectiveness are contradictory, at best. However, they seem to suggest that hay fever shots may be effective in reducing symptoms in many patients, while shots for food allergies are probably not. The critical question, as yet unanswered, is what potential consequences may affect your child in future years if he receives allergy shots. Apparently, the specialists in this field don't want to know the answer, because these desensitization shots have been given for decades, yet this question has never been adequately addressed.

The drugs commonly used in the treatment of allergic conditions, including asthma, have many potentially harmful and dangerous side effects. These antihistamines, steroid hormones, or xanthine derivatives are sold under trade names such as Aminophyllin, Aarane, Marax, Slophylline, Theodur, and Theobid, some to be taken orally and others via inhalers. All of them have side effects that may be merely annoying to your child but in many instances are dangerous. For example, steroid treatment of asthmatic children has been demonstrated to retard lung maturation and physical growth and to cause a higher incidence of cataracts in children receiving long-term steroid therapy.

I recommend that parents reject desensitization shots and drug therapy for their children unless the condition is life-threatening or until all of the alternatives have been explored. If you suspect that your child's illness is allergic in origin, look carefully for the potential source. You don't need a doctor to do this. First, consider all of the potential causes that exist in the child's environment, eliminate them one by one to the extent you can, and observe whether the symptoms are ameliorated or disappear. Begin an elimination diet in which suspect foods are eliminated from the diet one by one to determine whether one or more of the things he eats are responsible. The odds that you will discover the cause and solve the problem are substantially in your favor.

SEVERE ASTHMA REQUIRES MEDICAL HELP

While I am convinced that most allergic conditions do not required medical treatment, I don't want to minimize the need for medical attention for severe asthma and for immediate action in the event of a severe asthmatic attack. This is a potentially life-threatening condition, and it should be treated as such.

Unlike hay fever, which primarily affects the nasal passages, asthma is focused in the bronchial tubes. The allergen causes the small bronchial tubes to swell, a thick mucus is secreted, and the air passages become so clogged that breathing becomes difficult. In severe asthmatic attacks the patient wheezes, coughs, and gasps for breath, and the child's life may be at risk unless the condition is treated immediately. If this happens to your child, rush him to your doctor or, better still, to a hospital emergency room before the air passages become so clogged that he cannot get enough oxygen to survive. An injection of adrenaline will open up the airways, producing what amounts to a temporary miracle cure. Adrenaline, when used for this purpose, is an excellent drug that can be used practically with impunity.

Although asthma is usually allergic in origin, it is more baffling than the other allergic diseases because its onset is inconsistent and sometimes unrelated to causes that are specifically food or environmental allergens. Asthmatic attacks may be provoked by colds and other infections, by anxiety, by emotional upsets and other psychological conditions. Many parents are frustrated because their asthmatic child actually develops the ability to trigger an asthmatic attack by becoming emotionally upset over some disappointment or other event in his life. The frequency of attacks may also be related to exercise, climate, and even the season of the year.

As a parent who is in constant contact with your child, you are fully aware of his diet and the environmental conditions that surround him and are sensitive to his moods. Consequently, before you seek medical attention for any other than a life-threatening allergic condition, make a determined effort of your own to identify the cause. You are better qualified to do that than your doctor is. Only if your own efforts fail, and the illness persists or becomes life-threatening, need you consult a doctor.

DR. MENDELSOHN'S QUICK REFERENCE GUIDE TO ALLERGIES

As explained throughout this book, allergies should be suspect as the cause of a host of illnesses not typically associated with them. The appropriate action, when a disease is allergic in origin, is not to treat the symptoms with potentially dangerous drugs and desensitization shots but to identify and eliminate the allergen from the child's diet or environment. Parents are better qualified than doctors to undertake this mission because they know their child well, and have him under constant surveillance. If you suspect that your child's illness is allergic in origin, consider taking these steps:

1. Study every element of your child's environment, paying particular attention to the potential allergenic conditions and substances that are listed on page 214. If the symptoms of allergy are seasonal, occurring in the fall of the year, pollen should, of course, be the prime suspect.

2. If no environmental culprit is found, begin an elimination diet to determine whether your child is allergic to one or more specific foods. Eliminate food items that are most likely to be allergenic from the diet (see list on page 214) and observe whether the allergic symptoms disappear within 10 days or so. If they do, begin add-

ing each of these foods to his diet, one by one. If the symptoms reappear, you have identified one of the food items to which he is allergic. The reaction should occur within a couple of days. Repeat this process with the other food items until you have identified all of those that your child should avoid.

3. If you are unable to identify the allergen that is troubling your child, consult a human ecology allergist who can guide you in more sophisticated techniques for making this determination (see address on page 94). Only if that fails do I recommend consultation with a traditional allergist. If you do consult one, be extremely wary of scratch tests, desensitization injections, and drug treatments.

4. If your child's allergies produce a life-threatening condition, such as severe chronic asthma, a competent physician should be consulted in the event of a severe attack. This should not deter you from your efforts to identify the offending allergens, but it is essential to avoid life-threatening situations. If your asthmatic child has an attack so severe that breathing is dangerously inhibited, take him to your doctor or a hospital emergency room so that an injection of adrenaline can be administered at once.

18

The Child
Who Never
Sits Still

When your child reaches the toddler stage you may discover that he has more energy, is more active, and is less disciplined than most other kids of comparable age. At first you'll be pleased that he is outgoing and alert, not lethargic and withdrawn. Then, after chasing him day after day from one exploratory mishap to another, you may find that your reservoir of patience and stamina has been exhausted. That's when you'll begin to wonder whether his boundless energy is a blessing, after all. You may even worry that his behavior is abnormal; that he is "hyperactive" or a victim of "attention deficit disorder (ADD)," "learning disability (LD)," or "minimal brain damage (MBD)," all of which are so often diagnosed today.

My purpose in this chapter is to warn you of the hazards of making that diagnosis yourself, and of letting anyone else—doctor, teacher, or friend—do it for you. Once your child is given one of these labels there is a strong probability that he may be subjected to some unacceptable risks.

Professional counseling and drug treatment for children who exhibit exaggerated but perfectly normal developmental behavior has become almost epidemic in the United States. Largely because of pressure from school authorities, many American parents have lost faith in the legitimacy of their own decisions and in the accumulated wisdom of their parents, relatives, and friends. They've been led to believe that doctors and mental health professionals have the only answers to questions that previous generations answered quite effectively themselves.

If kids were made with cookie cutters, like the gingerbread man, norms could be set for your child's developmental behavior and the level of activity that he should display. Happily, they're not, with the result that no two children are precisely alike. That's frustrating for teachers, doctors, and every other professional who believes that everything in life should go by the book. It is not uncommon today for a child who is so active and inattentive that he gives his teacher fits to be diagnosed as "hyperactive" or "brain-damaged," treated with depressive chemicals, and isolated in the "learning lab" at school.

The possibility that your exceptionally active but perfectly normal child could be branded with one of these derogatory labels—none of which has a valid scientific definition—is not remote. The number of children who have suffered this fate has risen by 500,000 in the last five years. It could happen to your child if he displays some of these behaviors, which are on the checklists that psychologists use: doesn't always listen to directions; fidgets and won't sit still; daydreams in class; butts into situations that are none of his business; is slow getting ready for school; shows off when other children are around; or is more physically active than the other children in his class.

Your reaction to that list is probably the same as mine. I would begin to worry if a child didn't display most of those behaviors. Then I'd devote my attention to trying to diagnose why he is behaving like a vegetable! But when he does display them the mental health professionals are likely to give him drugs that often *do* turn him into something resembling a vegetable!

AVOID DRUGS FOR
BEHAVIOR MODIFICATION

If some of your child's behavior is more exaggerated and thus more annoying than that of other children you know, don't endanger him by exposing him to therapy or drugs. Instead, search for the environmental factors—at home, in school, or among his peers—that may be causing emotional problems. What pressures on your child are producing the behavior patterns that are unacceptable to his teachers and to you? Search also for dietary allergies that may be at the heart of his problems. Meanwhile, try to relieve some of the emotional pressure that his behavior is causing, provide strong emotional support at home, and let him know that he has you on his side when he encounters trouble outside your home.

In my experience, if it is carried out objectively and thoroughly, this approach usually works. Certainly, if it does, it is a desirable alternative to professional counseling that may cause your child to be labeled hyperactive, MBD, or ADD. If that happens, your child's school will probably place him in a special education program and assign him to a "learning laboratory," which will brand him as inferior among his peers. (In some schools the learning lab is derisively labeled—by the kids who aren't in it—as the "looney lab.")

I don't believe any child deserves that fate simply because he is harder to manage or harder to teach than the others in his class. This should concern you, but you should be even more concerned if psychoactive drugs, such as Ritalin or Cylert, are prescribed for your child.

Educators and doctors who label a child hyperactive or learning disabled, and then suggest treating him with chemicals, always defend their recommendations by asserting that it will improve the child's ability to learn. They know that you will respond to this more positively than to their true motivation, which is to drug your child into near-somnolence so he will be more manageable and less of a nuisance in the classroom.

No one has ever been able to demonstrate that drugs such as Cylert and Ritalin improve the academic performance of the children who take them. The major effect of Ritalin and similar drugs is on the short-term manageability of hyperkinetic behavior. The pupil is drugged to make life easier for his teacher, not to make it better and more productive for the child. If your child is the victim, the potential risks of these drugs is a high price to pay to make his teacher more comfortable.

DANGEROUS SIDE EFFECTS OF RITALIN

What are the risks to your child if he is put on Ritalin or a similar drug? First, there is ample evidence that they are prescribed inappropriately and administered carelessly and have side effects that are dangerous in themselves. Add to that the fact that they obviate the need and the incentive to discover what is really troubling your child, and you have a package that exemplifies contemporary medical practice and educational policy at their worst.

In the prescribing information for Ritalin that the manufacturer, Ciba-Geigy, supplied for the *Physician's Desk Reference*, the company acknowledges that it does not know how Ritalin works or how its effects relate to the condition of the central nervous system. It warns against the use of the drug in children under the age of six and admits that its long-term safety is unknown. It also notes that suppression of growth in those who take the drug has been noted in some cases and that there is some clinical evidence that it may provoke convulsive seizures in some patients.

The prescribing information then goes on to the potential side effects, which are so frightening that I will quote them directly from the book (the italicized phrases are mine):

> Nervousness and insomnia are the most common adverse reactions but are usually controlled by reducing dosage and omitting the drug in the afternoon and the evening. Other reactions include hypersensitivity (including skin rash), urticaria [*swollen, itching patches of skin*], fever, arthralgia, exfoliative dermatitis [*scaly patches of skin*], erythema multiforme [*an acute inflammatory skin disease*], with histopathological findings of necrotizing vasculitis [*destruction of the blood vessels*], and thrombocytopenic purpura [*a serious blood clotting disorder*], anorexia; nausea; dizziness; palpitations; headache; dyskinesia [*impairment of voluntary muscle movement*], drowsiness; blood pressure and pulse changes, both up and down; tachycardia [*rapid heartbeat*], angina [*spasmodic attacks of intense heart pain*]; cardiac arrhythmia [*irregular heartbeat*]; abdominal pain, weight loss during prolonged therapy.
>
> There have been rare reports of Tourette's syndrome. Toxic psychosis has been reported in patients taking this drug; leukopenia [*reduction in white blood cells*] and/or anemia; a few instances of scalp hair loss. In children, loss of appetite, abdominal pain, weight loss during prolonged therapy, insomnia, and tachycardia may occur more frequently; however, any of the other adverse reactions listed above may also occur.

This is the kind of information about a drug that the manufacturer is compelled by law to share with the doctors who will prescribe it. Unfortunately, there is no law requiring that the doctors who prescribe the drug share the information about its potentially damaging or fatal effects with you. That's why I have provided so much information about Ritalin, which applies, as well, to its counterparts.

If your child's teacher, school principal, counselor, or pediatrician attempts to pressure you into accepting chemical treatment for his behavior patterns, reject the advice out of hand. There is no benefit to your child that justifies the risks, nor can they be justified in order to spare his teacher the annoyance of having him talk out of turn or squirm in his seat.

LOOK FOR EMOTIONAL PRESSURES AS CAUSE

Don't accept a teacher's assessment of your child's behavioral shortcomings without investigating whether they may be the result of his or her interaction with him. Irreconcilable personality conflicts are not uncommon, and if one exists between your child and his teacher, the teacher may be the problem because he or she is not dealing equitably and sympathetically with your child. In that case the answer is to change teachers, not to use drugs to try to alter the behavior of her pupil.

While you are endeavoring to correct any conditions that are causing problems for your child at school, look for others that may be troubling him at home. If he is insecure because of stress among other family members, try to resolve those problems or at least avoid exposing him to the tensions that exist. If there are difficulties with his playmates or others outside your home, try to resolve those. Then turn your attention to the possibility that his hyperactive behavior may stem from allergies to food or other substances. There is substantial evidence that nutritional approaches may succeed in improving his emotional condition and behavior.

I must caution you that your pediatrician may not be sympathetic to this approach. The late Dr. Benjamin Feingold, the pioneer of dietary control of hyperactive behavior, encountered great skepticism from others in the medical profession. That's not surprising, because doctors chronically reject nonmedical solutions to problems they believe belong to them. Don't let that discourage you. Nervous system symptoms related to food hypersensitivity have been described by one observer after another for at least half a century. More recently, there has been a mass of clinical evidence that demonstrates that the Feingold diet does work with many children.

Dr. Feingold, who was chief of the allergy clinics of the Kaiser Foundation in California, zeroed in on chemical food additives—colorings, flavorings, preservatives, stabilizers, and others—as the principal contributors to hyperactive behavior. He recommended eliminating these chemicals from the diet by substituting natural foods for the highly processed items found in most American pantries and refrigerators. There is overwhelming clinical evidence that this approach is often successful.

Dr. Feingold's results have been duplicated by many others. Dr. William G. Crook, a pediatrician and allergist at the Children's Clinic in Jackson, Tennessee, reported on another study at a food allergy symposium. He said that hyperactivity was related to food allergy in about three-fourths of the cases in a study of more than 100 children who were overactive.

Dr. Crook observed precisely what Dr. Feingold had, and what many parents have, experienced: children can be helped by using elimination diets to identify offending foods. He identified milk and refined cane sugar as the leading culprits in a list that also included corn, wheat, eggs, soy, citrus, and other items.

If you have an overactive child with behavior problems, don't turn to drugs prescribed by your doctor until you have determined what success you have with food you can buy from your grocer!

QUESTION DIAGNOSIS
OF BRAIN DAMAGE

You should also be extremely wary of any suggestion that your child's behavior patterns stem from some form of brain damage or disorder. These conditions do exist in some children, of course, but the number is far fewer than the number of such cases that are diagnosed. Psychiatry is such an imprecise science, if it can be called a science, that its practitioners rarely agree on a diagnosis. Experiments have been conducted which show that psychologists and psychiatrists can be expected to agree with each other on a diagnosis only about 54 percent of the time. That's so close to the law of averages that you could consult a cabdriver and a carpenter and get the same result.

Nevertheless, on the basis of questionable diagnosis, your child may be recommended for psychotherapy if his behavior varies from what the mental health practitioner chooses to consider the "norm." Children who are correctly diagnosed as having brain or neurological damage or actual psychoses may benefit from treatment, of course. But short of that there is little evidence that psychological counseling helps and considerable evidence that it may actually aggravate a child's psychological/emotional problems.

The inadequacies of psychotherapy have been revealed repeatedly in follow-up studies of populations that have been exposed to psychiatric treatment. One well-known study points out that the spontaneous remission rate in patients with psychiatric conditions is 70 percent for both adults and children. Another study, reporting on a 20-year follow-up of patients at the University of Wisconsin, compared patients who were counseled with those who applied for but never received counseling. The most positive conclusion the study could reach was that *counseling seemed to do no harm*!

Another study of youths in Cambridge and Somerville, Massachusetts, was even less reassuring. It compared a group that had been counseled for five years, on a one-to-one basis, with a personal counselor, to another group that received no therapy at all. Almost without exception, psychological therapy appeared to have a *negative* effect on these youngsters in later life. Begun in 1939, this 30-year follow-up found a solid correlation between therapy and criminal behavior. More of the men who had received psychotherapy as youths were convicted of serious crimes and multiple crimes than those who had no treatment at all. Those who had the longest and most frequent contact with counselors had the highest incidence of antisocial and criminal behavior.

Finally, a 1980 review of 120 studies of psychotherapy for juvenile delinquents found that those who received counseling fared worse, in terms of subsequent behavior, than those who didn't. A report on this research in the Toronto *Globe & Mail* summed it up in this paragraph:

> If you want to stop a juvenile delinquent from robbing, raping, and clubbing people, don't send him to a social worker, a psychiatrist, a psychologist, a group home, a therapeutic community and don't make any efforts to counsel his family either. They all fail and some may even make him more violent than when he began.

There are, to be sure, some specific childhood mental and neurological disorders that stem from brain and neurological damage. Many of them are the consequence of medical interventions that I have discussed earlier in this book, e.g., cerebral palsy, Down's syndrome, Tourette's syndrome, autism, etc.

If your child is the victim of one of these conditions, professional help is appropriate, if for no other reason than to explore innovative treatment that may appear, e.g., the nutritional supplementation methods in the management of mongolism and other causes of mental retardation pioneered by Detroit's Henry Turkel, M.D., and Ruth Harrell, M.D., of Old Dominion University. However, if your child is suffering from this kind of condition—rather than behavior manifestations that simply make him more difficult to manage than other children— you'll know the difference. Your best course is to seek professional help when it is clearly needed, but avoid it if you are told that your child is suffering from a "learning disability," an "attention deficit disorder," or some other vaguely defined condition. The mental health professionals have yet to prove that any of these alleged disorders even exists!

19

Immunization against Disease: *A Medical Time Bomb?*

The greatest threat of childhood diseases lies in the dangerous and ineffectual efforts made to prevent them through mass immunization.

I know, as I write that line, that this concept is one that you may find difficult to accept. Immunizations have been so artfully and aggressively marketed that most parents believe them to be the "miracle" that has eliminated many once-feared diseases. Consequently, for anyone to oppose them borders on the foolhardy. For a pediatrician to attack what has become the "bread and butter" of pediatric practice is equivalent to a priest's denying the infallibility of the pope.

Knowing that, I can only hope that you will keep an open mind while I present my case. Much of what you have been led to believe about immunizations simply isn't true. I not only have grave misgivings about them; if I were to follow my deep convictions in writing this chapter, I would urge you to reject all inoculations for your child. I won't do that, because parents in about half the states have lost the right to make that choice. Doctors, not politicians, have successfully lobbied for laws that force parents to immunize their children as a prerequisite for admission to school.

Even in those states, though, you may be able to persuade your pediatrician to eliminate the pertussis (whooping cough) component from the DPT vaccine.

This immunization, which appears to be the most threatening of them all, is the subject of so much controversy that many doctors are becoming nervous about giving it, fearing malpractice suits. They should be nervous, because in a recent Chicago case a child damaged by a pertussis inoculation received a $5.5 million settlement award. If your doctor is in that state of mind, exploit his fear, because your child's health is at stake.

Although I administered them myself during my early years of practice, I have become a steadfast opponent of mass inoculations because of the myriad hazards they present. The subject is so vast and complex that it deserves a book of its own. Consequently, I must be content here with summarizing my objections to the fanatic zeal with which pediatricians blindly shoot foreign proteins into the body of your child without knowing what eventual damage they may cause.

Here is the core of my concern:

1. *There is no convincing scientific evidence that mass inoculations can be credited with eliminating any childhood disease*. While it is true that some once common childhood diseases have diminished or disappeared since inoculations were introduced. No one really knows why, although improved living conditions may be the reason. If immunizations were responsible for the disappearance of these diseases in the United States, one must ask why they disappeared simultaneously in Europe, where mass immunizations did not take place.

2. *It is commonly believed that the Salk vaccine was responsible for halting the polio epidemics that plagued American children in the 1940s and 1950s. If so, why did the epidemics also end in Europe, where polio vaccine was not so extensively used?* Of greater current relevance, why is the Sabin live virus vaccine still being administered to children when Dr. Jonas Salk, who pioneered the first vaccine, points out that Sabin vaccine is now causing most of the polio cases that appear. Con-

tinuing to force this vaccine on children is irrational medical behavior that simply confirms my contention that doctors consistently repeat their mistakes. With the polio vaccine we are witnessing a rerun of the medical reluctance to abandon the smallpox vaccination, which remained as the only source of smallpox-related deaths for three decades after the disease had disappeared.

Think of it! *For 30 years kids died from smallpox vaccinations even though no longer threatened by the disease.*

3. *There are significant risks associated with every immunization and numerous contraindications that may make it dangerous for the shots to be given to your child.* Yet doctors administer them routinely, usually without warning parents of the hazards and without determining whether the immunization is contraindicated for the child. No child should be immunized without making that determination, yet small armies of children are routinely lined up in clinics to receive a shot in the arm with no questions asked!

4. *While the myriad short-term hazards of most immunizations are known (but rarely explained), no one knows the long-term consequences of injecting foreign proteins into the body of your child.* Even more shocking is the fact that no one is making any structured effort to find out.

5. *There is a growing suspicion that immunization against relatively harmless childhood diseases may be responsible for the dramatic increase in autoimmune diseases since mass inoculations were introduced.* These are fearful diseases such as cancer, leukemia, rheumatoid arthritis, multiple sclerosis, Lou Gehrig's disease, lupus erythematosus, and the Guillain-Barre syndrome. An autoimmune disease can be explained simply as one in which the body's defense mechanisms cannot distinguish between foreign invaders and ordinary body tissues, with the consequence that the body begins to

destroy itself. Have we traded mumps and measles for cancer and leukemia?

I have emphasized these concerns because it is probable that your pediatrician will not advise you about them. At the 1982 Forum of the American Academy of Pediatrics (AAP), a resolution was proposed that would have helped insure that parents would be informed about the risks and benefits of immunizations. The resolution urged that the "AAP make available in clear, concise language information which a reasonable parent would want to know about the benefits and risks of routine immunizations, the risks of vaccine preventable diseases and the management of common adverse reactions to immunizations." Apparently the doctors assembled did not believe that "reasonable parents" were entitled to this kind of information because *they rejected the resolution*!

The bitter controversy over immunizations that is now raging within the medical profession has not escaped the attention of the media. Increasing numbers of parents are rejecting immunizations for their children and facing the legal consequences of doing so. Parents whose children have been permanently damaged by vaccines are no longer accepting this as fate but are filing malpractice suits against the manufacturers and the doctors who administered the vaccine. Some manufacturers have actually stopped making vaccines, and the lists of contraindications to their use are being expanded by the remaining manufacturers, year by year. Meanwhile, because routine immunizations that bring patients back for repeated office calls are the bread and butter of their specialty, pediatricians continue to defend them to the death.

The question parents should be asking is: Whose death?

As a parent, only you can decide whether to reject immunizations or risk accepting them for your child. Let me urge you, though—before your child is immunized—to arm yourself with the facts about the potential risks and benefits and demand that your pediatrician defend the immunizations that he recommends.

I will deal more fully with each of the most commonly administered immunizations in subsequent discussions of the diseases to which they are applied. If you decide that you don't want to have your child immunized, but your state laws say you must, write to me, and I may be able to offer suggestions on how you can regain your freedom of choice.

I am not going to try to cover all of the more obscure, life-threatening diseases in this book. However, in the remaining pages of this chapter I will describe the most common diseases, one or more of which may affect your child.

MUMPS

Mumps is a relatively innocuous viral disease, usually experienced in childhood, which causes swelling of one or both of the salivary glands (parotids), located just below and in front of the ears. Typical symptoms are a temperature of 100–104 degrees, appetite loss, headache, and back pain. The gland swelling usually begins to diminish after two or three days and is gone by the sixth or seventh day. However, one gland may become affected first, and the second as much as 10—12 days later. The infection of either side confers lifetime immunity.

Mumps does not require medical treatment. If your child contracts the disease, encourage him to stay in bed for two or three days, feed him a soft diet and a lot of fluids, and use ice packs to reduce the swelling. If his headache is severe, administer modest quantities of whiskey or acetaminophen. Give 10 drops of whiskey to a small baby and up to one-half teaspoon to a larger one. The dose can be repeated in one hour and once more in another hour, if needed.

Most children are immunized against mumps along

with measles and rubella in the MMR shot that is administered at about 15 months of age. Pediatricians defend this immunization with the argument that, although mumps is not a serious disease in children, if they do not gain immunity as children they may contract mumps as adults. In that event there is a possibility that adult males may contract orchitis, a condition in which the disease affects the testicles. In rare instances this can produce sterility.

If total sterility as a consequence of orchitis were a significant threat, and if the mumps immunization assured adult males that they would not contract it, I would be among those doctors who urge immunization. I'm not, because their argument makes no sense. Orchitis rarely causes sterility, and when it does, because only one testicle is usually affected, the sperm production capacity of the unaffected testicle could repopulate the world! And that's not all. No one knows whether the mumps vaccination confers an immunity that lasts into the adult years. Consequently, there is an open question whether, when your child is immunized against mumps at 15 months and escapes this disease in childhood, he may suffer more serious consequences when he contracts it as an adult.

If the mumps immunization is given to protect adult males from orchitis, not to prevent children from getting mumps, it would seem reasonable to administer it only to those males who haven't developed natural immunity by the time they reach puberty. They would then be more certain of protection as adults. All girls and countless boys would thus avoid the potential consequences of a hazardous vaccine.

You won't find pediatricians advertising them, but the side effects of the mumps vaccine can be severe. In some children it causes allergic reactions such as rash, itching, and bruising. It may also expose them to the effects of central nervous system involvement, including febrile seizures, unilateral nerve deafness, and encephalitis. The risks are minimal, true, but why should your child endure them at all to avoid an innocuous disease in childhood at the risk of contracting a more serious one as an adult?

MEASLES

Measles, also called rubeola or "English measles," is a contagious viral disease that can be contracted by touching an object used by an infected person. At the onset the victim feels tired, has a slight fever and pains in the head and back. His eyes redden and he may be sensitive to light. The fever rises until about the third or fourth day, when it reaches 103–104 degrees. Sometimes small white spots can be seen inside the mouth, and a rash of small pink spots appears below the hairline and behind the ears. This rash spreads downward to cover the body in about 36 hours. The pink spots may run together but fade away in about three or four days. Measles is contagious for seven or eight days, beginning three or four days before the rash appears. Consequently, if one of your children contracts the disease, the others probably will have been exposed to it before you know the first child is sick.

No treatment is required for measles other than bed rest, fluids to combat possible dehydration from fever, and calamine lotion or cornstarch baths to relieve the itching. If the child suffers from photophobia, the blinds in his bedroom should be lowered to darken the room. However, contrary to the popular myth, there is no danger of permanent blindness from this disease.

A vaccine to prevent measles is another element of the MMR inoculation given in early childhood. Doctors maintain that the inoculation is necessary to prevent measles encephalitis, which they say occurs about once in 1,000 cases. After decades of experience with measles, I question this statistic, and so do many other pediatricians. The incidence of 1/1000 may be accurate for children who live in conditions of poverty and malnutrition, but in the middle- and upper-income brackets, if one excludes simple sleepiness from the measles itself, the incidence of true encephalitis is probably more like 1/10,000 or 1/100,000.

After frightening you with the unlikely possibility of measles encephalitis, your doctor can rarely be counted on to tell you of the dangers associated with the vaccine he uses to prevent it. The measles vaccine is associated with encephalopathy and with a series of other complications such as SSPE (subacute sclerosing panencephalitis), which causes hardening of the brain and is invariably fatal.

Other neurologic and sometimes fatal conditions associated with the measles vaccine include ataxia (inability to coordinate muscle movements), mental retardation, aseptic meningitis, seizure disorders, and hemiparesis (paralysis affecting one side of the body). Secondary complications associated with the vaccine may be even more frightening. They include encephalitis, subacute sclerosing panencephalitis, multiple sclerosis, toxic epidermal necrolysis, anaphylactic shock, Reye's syndrome, Guillain-Barre syndrome, blood clotting disorders, juvenile-onset diabetes, and even a relationship with Hodgkin's disease and cancer.

I would consider the risks associated with measles vaccination unacceptable even if there were convincing evidence that the vaccine works. There isn't. While there has been a decline in the incidence of the disease, it began long before the vaccine was introduced. In 1958 there were about 800,000 cases of measles in the United States, but by 1962—the year *before* a vaccine appeared—the number of cases had dropped by 300,000. During the next four years, while children were being vaccinated with an ineffective and now abandoned "killer virus" vaccine, the number of cases dropped another 300,000. In 1900 there were 13.3 measles deaths per 100,000 population. By 1955, before the first measles shot, the death rate had declined 97.7 percent to only 0.03 deaths per 100,000.

Those numbers alone are dramatic evidence that measles was disappearing before the vaccine was introduced. If you fail to find them sufficiently convincing, consider this: in a 1978 survey of 30 states, more than half of the children who contracted measles had been adequately vaccinated. Moreover, according to the World Health Organization, the chances are about 15 times greater that measles will be contracted by those vaccinated for them than by those who are not.

"Why," you may ask, "in the face of these facts, do doctors continue to give the shots?" The answer may lie in an episode that occurred in California 14 years after the measles vaccine was introduced. Los Angeles suffered a severe measles epidemic during that year, and parents were urged to vaccinate all children six months of age and older—despite a Public Health warning that vaccinating children below the age of one year was useless and potentially harmful.

Although Los Angeles doctors responded by routinely shooting measles vaccine into every kid they could get their hands on, several local physicians familiar with the suspected problems of immunologic failure and "slow virus" dangers chose not to vaccinate their own infant children. Unlike their patients, who weren't told, they realized that "slow viruses" found in all live vaccines, and particularly in the measles vaccine, can hide in human tissue for years. They may emerge later in the form of encephalitis, multiple sclerosis, and as potential seeds for the development and growth of cancer.

One Los Angeles physician who refused to vaccinate his own 7-month-old-baby said: "I'm worried about what happens when the vaccine virus may not only offer little protection against measles but may also stay around in the body, working in a way we don't know much about." His concern about the possibility of these consequences for his own child, however, did not cause him to stop vaccinating his infant patients. He rationalized this contradictory behavior with the comment that "As a parent, I have the *luxury* of making a choice for my child. As a physician... legally and professionally I have to accept the recommendations of the profession, which is what we also had to do with the whole Swine flu-business."

Perhaps it is time that lay parents and their children are granted the same luxury that doctors and their children enjoy.

RUBELLA

Commonly known as "German measles," rubella is a non-threatening disease in children that does not require medical treatment. The initial symptoms are fever and a slight cold, accompanied by a sore throat. You know it is something more when a rash appears on the face and scalp and spreads to the arms and body. The spots do not run together as they do with measles, and they usually fade away after two or three days. The victim should be encouraged to rest and be given adequate fluids, but no other treatment is needed.

The threat posed by rubella is the possibility that it may cause damage to the fetus if a woman contracts the disease during the first trimester of pregnancy. This fear is used to justify the immunization of all children, boys and girls, as part of the MMR inoculation. The merits of this vaccine are questionable for essentially the same reasons that apply to mumps inoculations. There is no need to protect children from this harmless disease, so the adverse reactions to the vaccine are unacceptable in terms of benefit to the child. They can include arthritis, arthralgia (painful joints), and polyneuritis, which produces pain, numbness, or tingling in the peripheral nerves. While these symptoms are usually temporary, they may last for several months and may not occur until as long as two months after the vaccination. Because of that time lapse, parents may not identify the cause when these symptoms appear in their vaccinated child.

The greater danger of rubella vaccination is the possibility that it may deny expectant mothers the protection of natural immunity from the disease. By preventing rubella in childhood, immunization may actually increase the threat that women will contract rubella during their childbearing years. My concern on this score is shared by many other doctors. In Connecticut a group of doctors, led by two eminent epidemiologists, have actually succeeded in getting rubella stricken from the list of legally required immunizations.

Study after study has demonstrated that many women immunized against rubella as children lack evidence of immunity in blood tests given during their adolescent years. Other tests have shown a high vaccine failure rate in children given rubella, measles, and mumps shots, either separately or in combined form. Finally, the crucial question yet to be answered is whether vaccine-induced immunity is as effective and long-lasting as immunity from the natural disease of rubella. A large proportion of children show no evidence of immunity in blood tests given only four or five years after rubella vaccination.

The significance of this is both obvious and frightening. Rubella is a nonthreatening disease in childhood, and it confers natural immunity to those who contract it so they will not get it again as adults. Prior to the time that doctors began giving rubella vaccinations an estimated 85 percent of adults were naturally immune to the disease.

Today, because of immunization, the vast majority of women never acquire natural immunity. If their vaccine-induced immunity wears off, they may contract rubella while they are pregnant, with resulting damage to their unborn children.

Being a skeptical soul, I have always believed that the most reliable way to determine what people really believe is to observe what they do, not what they say. If the greatest threat of rubella is not to children, but to the fetus yet unborn, pregnant women should be protected against rubella by making certain that their obstetricians won't give them the disease. Yet, in a California survey reported in the *Journal of the American Medical*

Association, more than 90 percent of the obstetrician-gynecologists refused to be vaccinated. If doctors themselves are afraid of the vaccine, why on earth should the law require that you and other parents allow them to administer it to your kids?

WHOOPING COUGH

Whooping cough (pertussis) is an extremely contagious bacterial disease that is usually transmitted through the air by an infected person. The incubation period is 7–14 days. The initial symptoms are indistinguishable from those of a common cold: a runny nose, sneezing, listlessness and loss of appetite, some tearing in the eyes, and sometimes a mild fever.

As the disease progresses, the victim develops a severe cough at night. Later it appears during the day, as well. Within a week to 10 days after the first symptoms appear the cough will become paroxysmal. The child may cough a dozen times with each breath, and his face may darken to a bluish or purple hue. Each coughing bout ends with a whooping intake of breath, which accounts for the popular name for the disease. Vomiting is often an additional symptom of the disease.

Whooping cough can strike within any age group, but more than half of all victims are below two years of age. It can be serious and even life-threatening, particularly in infants. Infected persons can transmit the disease to others for about a month after the appearance of the initial symptoms, so it is important that they be isolated, especially from other children.

If your child contracts whooping cough, there is no specific treatment that your doctor can provide, nor is there any you can apply at home, other than to encourage your child to rest and to provide comfort and consolation. Cough suppressants are sometimes used, but they rarely help very much and I don't recommend them. However, if an infant contracts the disease, you should consult a doctor because hospital care may be required. The primary threats to babies are exhaustion from coughing and pneumonia. Very young infants have even been known to suffer cracked ribs from the severe coughing bouts.

Immunization against pertussis is given along with vaccines for diphtheria and tetanus in the DPT inoculation. Although the vaccine has been used for decades, it is one of the most controversial of immunizations. Doubts persist about its effectiveness, and many doctors share my concern that the potentially damaging side effects of the vaccine may outweigh the alleged benefits.

Dr. Gordon T. Stewart, head of the department of community medicine at the University of Glasgow, Scotland, is one of the most vigorous critics of the pertussis vaccine. He says he supported the inoculation before 1974 but then began to observe outbreaks of pertussis in children who had been vaccinated. "Now, in Glasgow," he says, "30 percent of our whooping cough cases are occurring in vaccinated patients. This leads me to believe that the vaccine is not all that protective."

As in the case with other infectious diseases, mortality had begun to decline before the vaccine became available. The vaccine was not introduced until about 1936, but mortality from the disease had already been declining steadily since 1900 or earlier. According to Stewart, "the decline in pertussis mortality was 80 percent before the vaccine was ever used." He shares my view that the key factor in controlling whooping cough is probably not the vaccine but improvement in the living conditions of potential victims.

Others in the profession do not deal kindly with doctors who raise questions about their cherished vaccines. In 1982 I appeared in a one-hour NBC television documentary devoted to the pertussis vaccine controversy and commented that "the danger [from the vaccine] is far greater than any doctors here have ever been willing to admit." In July 1982, the *Journal of the American Medical Association*, in a bitter attack on the program, charged that the network chose dubious 'experts' to badmouth the vaccine and endowed them with false credentials." It then proceeded to attack my credentials.

I don't feel any compulsion to defend myself from the American Medical Association which, over the years, has had to spend an inordinate portion of its budget in its own self-defense. It is instructive, however, to read what that same issue of the *AMA Journal* had to say about the risks of pertussis vaccine. I'll cite what they had to say and let you judge whether it is inappropriate for me to raise questions about its use. For starters, *JAMA* said this:

> To health professionals, of course, the dangers of DPT are nothing new. The D and T components, which were given long before the P was added in the late 1940s, are partially purified toxoids considered to carry little risk. The whole-cell P component, consisting of 4 units of protective pertussis antigen per 0.5 ml of DPT is universally acknowledged to be *relatively crude and toxic, and the advent of a safer version is eagerly awaited* (italics mine).
>
> Almost from the inception of widespread DPT immunization, severe reactions have been reported, beginning with Byers's and Moll's study of vaccine-associated encephalopathy in 1948. The incidence of such reactions has not been firmly established. It does seem fairly certain that vaccine-associated seizures, unusual as they are, are considerably more common than brain damage or residual impairment secondary to such seizures.

It is obvious from this statement that the American Medical Association does not deny that pertussis vaccine is hazardous, with the potential of frightening side effects. Their concern is over the fact that media attention is making the recipients of the vaccine aware of the risks!

If it is improper for a doctor to share with his patients his knowledge of the risks of immunization, I plead guilty to the charge. The common side effects of the pertussis vaccine, acknowledged by *JAMA*, are fever, crying bouts, a shocklike state, and local skin effects such as swelling, redness, and pain. Less frequent but more serious side effects include convulsions and permanent brain damage resulting in mental retardation. The vaccine has also been linked to Sudden Infant Death Syndrome (SIDS). In 1978–79, during an expansion of the Tennessee childhood immunization program, eight cases of SIDS were reported immediately following routine DPT immunization.

Estimates of the number of those vaccinated with the pertussis vaccine who are protected from the disease range from 50 percent to 80 percent. According to *JAMA*, reported cases of whooping cough in the United States total an average of 1,000–3,000 per year and deaths 5–20 per year.

My question is: Does it make sense to expose millions of children each year to the potential hazards of the vaccine in order to provide them with dubious protection against a disease that is so rarely seen?

DIPHTHERIA

Although it was one of the most feared of childhood diseases in grandma's day, diphtheria has now almost disappeared. Only five cases were reported in the United States in 1980. Most doctors insist that the decline is due to immunization with the DPT vaccine, but there is ample evidence that the incidence of diphtheria was already diminishing before a vaccine became available.

Diphtheria is a highly contagious bacterial disease that is spread by the coughing and sneezing of infected persons or by handling items that they have touched. The incubation period for the disease is two to five days, and the first symptoms are a sore throat, headache, nausea, coughing, and a fever of 100–104 degrees. As the disease progresses, dirty-white patches can be observed on the tonsils and in the throat. They cause swelling in the throat and larnyx that makes swallowing difficult and, in severe cases, may obstruct breathing to the point that the victim chokes to death. The disease requires medical attention and can be treated with antibiotics such as penicillin or erythromycin.

Today your child has about as much chance of contracting diphtheria as he does of being bitten by a cobra. Yet millions of children are immunized against it with repeated injections at 2, 4, 6 and 18 months and then given a booster shot when they enter school. This despite evidence over more than a dozen years from rare outbreaks of the disease that children who have been immunized fare no better than those who have not. During a 1969 outbreak of diphtheria in Chicago the city board of health reported that 4 of the 16 victims had been fully immunized against the disease and 5 others had received one or more doses of the vaccine. Two of the latter showed evidence of full immunity. A report on another outbreak in which three people died revealed that one of the fatal cases and 14 of 23 carriers had been fully immunized.

Episodes such as these shatter the argument that immunization can be credited with eliminating diphtheria or any of the other once common childhood diseases. If immunization deserved the credit, how do its defenders explain this? Only about half the states have legal requirements for immunization against infectious diseases, and the percentage of children immunized varies from state to state. As a consequence, tens of thousands —perhaps millions—of children in areas where medical services are limited and pediatricians almost nonexistent were never immunized against infectious diseases and therefore should be vulnerable to them. Yet the incidence of infectious diseases does not correlate in any respect with whether a state has legally mandated mass immunization or not.

In view of the rarity of the disease, the effective antibiotic treatment now available, the questionable effectiveness of the vaccine, the multimillion-dollar annual cost of administering it, and the ever-present potential for harmful, long-term effects from this or any other vaccine, I consider continued mass immunization against diphtheria indefensible. I grant that no significant harmful effects from the vaccine have been identified, but that doesn't mean they aren't there. In the half-century that the vaccine has been used no research has ever been undertaken to determine what the long-term effects of the vaccine may be!

CHICKEN POX

This is my favorite childhood disease, first because it is relatively innocuous and second because it is one of the few for which no pharmaceutical manufacturer has yet marketed a vaccine. That second reason may be short-lived, though, because as this is written there are reports that a chicken pox vaccine soon may appear.

Chicken pox is a communicable viral infection that is very common in children. The first signs of the disease are usually a slight fever, headache, backache, and loss of appetite.

After a day or two, small red spots appear, and within a few hours they enlarge and become blisters. Ultimately a scab forms that peels off, usually within a week or two. This process is accompanied by severe itching, and the child should be encouraged not to scratch the sores. Calamine lotion may be applied, or cornstarch baths given, to relieve the itching.

It is not necessary to seek medical treatment for chicken pox. The patient should be encouraged to rest and to drink a lot of fluids to prevent dehydration from the fever.

The incubation period for chicken pox is from two to three weeks, and the disease is contagious for about two weeks, beginning two days after the rash appears. The child should be isolated during this period to avoid spreading the disease to others.

SCARLET FEVER

Scarlet fever is another example of a once feared disease that has virtually disappeared. If a vaccine had ever been developed for it, doctors would undoubtedly credit that with the elimination of the disease. Since there is no vaccine, they give the credit to penicillin, despite the fact that the disease was already disappearing before the first antibiotics appeared. In all probability, as with other diseases, the true reason for its waning incidence is improved living conditions and better nutrition.

The disease got its name from the red rash that covers the body of victims. It is caused by a streptococcus infection, and the initial symptoms are vomiting, headache, a swelling of the lymph nodes in the neck, and a fever of 101–105 degrees. The disease usually affects children between the ages of two and eight, and the rash that accompanies it fades in about a week. If your child contracts scarlet fever, which is most unlikely, you need not be alarmed because it is no more dangerous than a strep throat infection. It will disappear by itself, but if you take your child to a doctor, he is likely to prescribe an antibiotic that your child really doesn't need.

MENINGITIS

One of the appalling inconsistencies of contemporary medical practice is the tendency of doctors to overtreat the diseases that don't require treatment, and miss the diagnosis in diseases like meningitis that deserve all of the skill they have to offer. This disease is an inflammation of the membranes that cover the brain and the spinal cord, called the *meninges*. The symptoms may include a stiff neck (but not necessarily), a persistent headache, vomiting, fever, and convulsions in infants. Bacterial, viral, and fungal infections can cause the disease. One of the bacterial types is particularly contagious because the bacteria are found in the throat as well as in the cerebrospinal fluid.

Meningitis is amenable to treatment, but early diagnosis is essential. Doctors often miss the diagnosis because they fail to take the mother seriously when she reports significant changes in her child's behavior. Many also fail to give serious consideration to the possibility of meningitis unless the child has a stiff neck.

Potential consequences of failure to diagnose and treat meningitis properly are mental retardation and death. If your child has an unexplained fever for three or four days, accompanied by drowsiness, vomiting, *a shrill cry*, and possibly a stiff neck, it is time to suspect meningitis. Some of these symptoms are also present with influenza. You can distinguish meningitis by the last two, particularly the shrill cry. If your child has this, insist that your doctor perform the appropriate tests, which may include a spinal tap. In that event, if he doesn't find the spinal canal on the first or second attempt, tell him to stop trying and call another doctor.

Antibiotics have reduced mortality from this dread disease from 95 percent to 5 percent. That's why correct, early diagnosis of the disease is a matter of life or death.

TUBERCULOSIS

Parents should have the right to assume, and most do assume, that the tests their doctor gives their child will produce an accurate result. The tuberculin skin test is but one example of a medical test procedure in which that is definitely not the case. Even the American Academy of Pediatrics, which rarely has anything negative to say about procedures that its members routinely employ, has issued a policy statement that is critical of this test. According to the statement,

> Several recent studies have cast doubt on the sensitivity of some screening tests for tuberculosis. Indeed a panel assembled by the Bureau of Biologics has recommended to manufacturers that each lot be tested in 50 known positive patients to assure that preparations that are marketed are potent enough to identify everyone with active tuberculosis. However, since many of these studies have not been conducted in a randomized, double-blind fashion and/or have included many simultaneously administered skin tests (thus the possibility of suppression of reactions), interpretation of the tests is difficult.

The statement concludes, "Screening tests for tuberculosis are not perfect, and physicians must be aware of the possibility that some false negative as well as positive reactions may be obtained."

In short, your child may have tuberculosis, even though there is a negative reading on his tuberculin test. Or he may not have it but display a positive skin test that says he does. With many doctors, this can lead to some devastating consequences. Almost certainly, if this happens to your child, he will be exposed to needless and hazardous radiation from one or more x-rays of his chest. The doctor may then place him on dangerous drugs such as isoniazid for months or years "to prevent the development of tuberculosis." Even the AMA has recognized that doctors have indiscriminately overprescribed isoniazid. That's shameful, because of the drug's long list of side effects on the nervous system, gastrointestinal system, blood, bone marrow, skin, and endocrine glands. Also not to be overlooked is the danger that your child may become a pariah in your neighborhood because of the lingering fear of this infectious disease.

I am convinced that the potential consequences of a positive tuberculin skin test are more dangerous than the threat of the disease. I believe parents should reject the test unless they have specific knowledge that their child has been in contact with someone who has the disease.

SUDDEN INFANT DEATH SYNDROME (SIDS)

The dreadful possibility that they may awaken some morning to find their baby dead in his crib is a fear that lurks in the minds of many parents. Medical science has yet to pinpoint the cause of SIDS, but the most popular explanation among researchers appears to be that the central nervous system is somehow affected so that the involuntary act of breathing is suppressed.

That is a logical explanation, but it leaves unanswered the question: What caused the malfunction in the central nervous system? My suspicion, which is shared by others in my profession, is that the nearly 10,000 SIDS deaths that occur in the United States each year are related to one or more of the vaccines that are routinely given children. The pertussis vaccine is the most likely villain, but it could also be one or more of the others.

Dr. William Torch, of the University of Nevada School of Medicine at Reno, has issued a report suggesting that the DPT shot may be responsible for SIDS cases. He found that two-thirds of 103 children who died of SIDS had been immunized with DPT vaccine in the three weeks before their deaths, many dying within a day after getting the shot. He asserts that this was not mere coincidence, concluding that a "causal relationship is suggested" in at least some cases of DPT vaccine and crib death. Also on record are the Tennessee deaths, referred to earlier. In that case the manufacturer of the vaccine, following intervention by the U.S. surgeon general, recalled all unused doses of this batch of vaccine.

More recently, in 1983, the department of pediatrics

of the UCLA School of Medicine and the Los Angeles County health department reported another disturbing study of 145 SIDS victims. Of this number, 53 had received DPT immunizations in close proximity to their deaths. Twenty-seven died within 28 days of being immunized, 17 of those within a week after receiving the DPT shot, and six within 24 hours of receiving it. The researchers concluded that these findings "further substantiate a possible association" between DPT shots and SIDS.

Expectant mothers who are concerned about SIDS should bear in mind the importance of breastfeeding to avoid this and other serious ailments. There is evidence that breastfed babies are less susceptible to allergies, respiratory disease, gastroenteritis, hypocalcemia, obesity, multiple sclerosis, and SIDS. One study of the scientific literature about SIDS concluded that "Breastfeeding can be seen as a common block to the myriad of pathways to SIDS."

POLIOMYELITIS

No one who lived through the 1940s and saw photos of children in iron lungs, saw a President of the United States confined to his wheelchair by this dread disease, and was forbidden to use public beaches for fear of catching polio can forget the fear that prevailed at the time. Polio is virtually nonexistent today, but much of that fear persists, and there is a popular belief that immunization can be credited with eliminating the disease. That's not surprising, considering the high-powered campaign that promoted the vaccine, but the fact is that no credible scientific evidence exists that the vaccine caused polio to disappear. As noted earlier, it also disappeared in other parts of the world where the vaccine was not so extensively used.

What is important to parents of this generation is the evidence that points to mass inoculation against polio as the cause of most remaining cases of the disease. In September 1977 Jonas Salk, the developer of the killed polio virus vaccine, testified along with other scientists to that effect. He said that most of the handful of polio cases which had occurred in the U.S. since the early 1970s probably were the by-product of the live polio vaccine that is in standard use in the United States. In Finland and Sweden there have been no cases of polio in more than a decade, but in those countries the killed virus vaccine is used almost exclusively.

Meanwhile, there is an ongoing debate among the immunologists regarding the relative risks of killed virus vs. live virus vaccine. Supporters of the killed virus vaccine maintain that it is the presence of live virus organisms in the other product that is responsible for the polio cases that occasionally appear. Supporters of the live virus type argue that the killed virus vaccine offers inadequate protection and actually increases the susceptibility of those vaccinated to the disease.

This affords me a rare opportunity to be comfortably neutral. I believe that both factions are right and that use of either of the vaccines will increase, not diminish, the possibility that your child will contract the disease.

In short, it appears that the most effective way to protect your child from polio is to make sure that he doesn't get the vaccine!

INFECTIOUS MONONUCLEOSIS

The symptoms of infectious mononucleosis resemble those of the common cold or influenza, so in its early stages it is not likely to be suspected or diagnosed. It usually affects children and young adults, and if your child is the victim, he will display fever, swollen glands, a sore throat, weakness, and fatigue. As the disease progresses, the symptoms may also include abdominal pain, nausea, headaches, chest pain, coughing, and several other less common symptoms.

If your child has these symptoms and they persist beyond the normal course of a common cold, he should see a doctor. If the doctor suspects mononucleosis, he will probably order a blood test, which will usually, although not always, determine whether mononucleosis is present. The disease usually runs its course in one to three weeks, but in extreme cases it may persist for weeks or even months.

The fact that mononucleosis, in its early stages, cannot be distinguished from other ailments such as the common cold need not concern you because there is no specific drug treatment for the disease. The treatment is what you would be giving your child in any event—bed rest and liberal fluids. Some doctors prescribe adrenal steroids such as prednisone for mononucleosis, but I believe they should be avoided except in extreme cases of the disease. They have serious side effects, as described in Chapter 17.

20

Hospitals:
Where Patients Go
to Get Sick!

Throughout this book I have tried to help you identify illnesses that require medical treatment and to alert you to forms of treatment that may be more dangerous than the disease that is being treated. One final admonition is required: *Don't allow your child to be admitted to a hospital unless his condition is so serious that his life is in danger.*

Relatively few childhood ailments require hospitalization, but many children are hospitalized needlessly simply because it is more convenient (and more profitable) for their doctor. Most illnesses and accidental injuries can be treated as effectively in the emergency room, a doctor's office, or an outpatient clinic, without hospitalization, and your child will usually receive better, safer care at home.

There are two major categories of disease that are unique to those who seek medical treatment and particularly to those who are hospitalized as a result. You may never have heard of either of them, because their names are rarely used by doctors in the presence of their patients. Why? Because *iatrogenic* is the term applied to illnesses and injuries *caused* by doctors, and *nosocomial* is the term used to describe infections acquired by patients after they enter a hospital. Both constitute major threats to your child if you permit him to be hospitalized.

About 2 million Americans are admitted to hospitals each year for the treatment of one ailment and end up with another. The illnesses they acquire in the hospital prove to be fatal to as many as 20,000 of them. The number who contract nosocomial illnesses equals about 5 percent of hospital admissions. In other words, if your child enters the hospital with one disease, the chances are 1 in 20 that he will contract another one before he is released. Moreover, there is a real possibility that before he is released the disease he acquired in the hospital may kill him. If his admission to the hospital was for a life-threatening condition, that may be an acceptable risk, but if his admission was not essential, it is certainly a risk your child should avoid.

These risks are rarely revealed in publications that patients read, but doctors are well aware of them from reports published in their medical journals. One such report in the *Journal of the American Medical Association* in 1978 had this to say about the mortality and cost of nosocomial infections:

> Hospital patients with nosocomial bacteremia [bacterial blood infections] and matched hospital control patients without this infection were used to determine the excess hospital costs and mortality attributed to nosocomial bacteremias. Mortality was 14 times greater in patients with nosocomial bacteremia than in matched numbers of the control group with the same primary diagnoses. An itemized cost analysis, based on 81 case-control pairs, showed an average excess of approximately $3,600 in direct hospital costs for patients who had nosocomial bacteremias.

The hospital-acquired infections caused the average patient to remain in the hospital for 14 additional days. At today's skyrocketing daily hospital rates, that $3,600 figure would probably be doubled or tripled.

RESPIRATORY ILLNESSES CONTRACTED IN HOSPITALS

A study done six years ago in a hospital pediatric ward revealed that *one-sixth of the children at risk acquired respiratory illnesses while in the hospital.* There have also been countless instances of epidemic disease among hospitalized children. In 1979, for example, two children died and three others suffered permanent paralysis or brain damage during an outbreak of meningitis in a Florida hospital nursery. In the Florida epidemic, and in most of the others, the outbreak was traced to the *failure of medical personnel to wash their hands!*

It is well over a century since a Hungarian physician, Ignaz Semmelweis, discovered that deaths from "childbirth fever" resulted from the failure of medical students to wash their hands. His findings were generally rejected by others in his profession, and he was driven into obscurity, finally to die in an asylum—presumably of a hospital-caused infection. Apparently medical personnel are slow learners, because many of them still haven't gotten his message today.

In 1981 a study was conducted for more than two months in the intensive care units of a private hospital and a university-affiliated teaching hospital. Researchers observed the hand-washing habits of doctors, nurses, and other medical personnel. The medical personnel washed up between patients only 41 percent of the time in the teaching hospital and only 28 percent of the time in the private hospital. Doctors were the worst offenders. They washed their hands only 28 percent of the time in the teaching hospital and 14 percent of the time in the private hospital.

I'm dwelling on this because I want to disabuse you of the notion—held by most people—that a hospital is a hygienic, virtually sterile sanctuary for your child. In fact, as the studies indicate, the sanitary practices of the medical personnel are often abominable, and the hospital itself is probably the most germ-laden facility in town. If you can't avoid it, you can at least be forewarned and demand that appropriate sanitary precautions be taken for your child.

The threat of iatrogenic illness also mounts in the hospital, because doctors are so strongly motivated by instinct, training, and unwarranted fear of malpractice suits to employ all of the medical technology available to them, even when it is of dubious value in diagnosis and treatment. Everything your doctor does presents an added risk for your child. Every needle he inserts makes a new pathway into the body for infectious organisms; every drug he administers yields the possibility of harmful side effects; every X-ray he orders holds the possibility of causing radiation-induced damage to your child in his later years.

Countless studies have shown that iatrogenic illness contracted in hospitals is not an isolated phenomenon. In one such study 815 consecutive patients in the general medical service of a university hospital were evaluated. More than a third of them—36 percent—were found to have a disease condition caused by something done to them by a physician. A total of 165 patients had one physician-caused condition, and 125 of them had from two to seven iatrogenic conditions. These included heart and lung complications, infections or inflammation, gastrointestinal problems, nerve damage, allergic reactions, bleeding, and metabolic complications.

For at least two decades other studies have reported similar results. In 1963 a study of 1,000 patients admitted to a university hospital during an eight-month period revealed that 20 percent of them had acquired an iatrogenic disease during their stay. Fifty-one percent of the victims had complications due to the administration of drugs, and 24 percent were the aftermaths of diagnostic or therapeutic procedures. Illnesses related to preexisting complications, nursing errors, and the untoward effects of surgery were excluded from the study, or the numbers would have been even more shocking.

EMOTIONAL IMPACT OF HOSPITALIZATION

The hazards of hospitalization for the young child are not limited to the physical risks. There may be damaging psychological and emotional consequences as well. For a youngster, mere separation from his mother and family for any period of time can be a traumatic experience. When that separation is associated with the awesome atmosphere of the hospital setting, the experience is almost inevitably a frightening one for a child.

The emotional and psychological damage from such an experience is not always transient. The possibility of long-term effects is substantial, as was noted in *Pediatrics*, the Journal of the American Academy of Pediatrics in November 1979:

> When a young child must be hospitalized, the effects of the experience can be very detrimental. Several studies have indicated that these effects may evidence themselves as behavior disturbances, regressed development, retarded recovery, and the like. Two studies from Britain provide striking evidence that a hospital admission of greater than one week's duration, or repeated short admissions before the age of five years, are associated with an increased incidence of behavior disturbances at age 10 years and into adolescence.

My intention in this chapter has been to alert you to the risks your child will face if you permit him to be admitted to a hospital. I also realize, though, that one of these days your pediatrician may insist on hospitalizing your child, and you will need to know how to respond! What should you do if that day arrives?

First, demand that your doctor prove to your satisfaction that the things he plans to do in the hospital can't be done in his office, in an outpatient facility, or at home.

Except in life-threatening situations, which may require sophisticated medical monitoring around the clock, there is virtually no diagnostic procedure that can't be done on an outpatient basis and virtually no illness that can't be treated by an informed parent at home.

Second, if the admission is for a surgical procedure, make certain that the surgery is really required and that it can't be provided on an outpatient basis, with the aftercare provided at home. As I have indicated in other chapters, most of the surgery performed on children is unnecessary, and most of that which is indicated can be performed safely and adequately without hospitalizing the child. Why risk hospitalizing him for one ailment at the risk of giving him another?

Third, if hospitalization is unavoidable, don't permit your child to spend one hour there alone. When you can't be with him yourself, make certain that some other familiar face and concerned observer is at hand. Familiarize yourself with the medications and treatments he is supposed to be given and watch the medical personnel like a hawk so they don't make any mistakes. They're human and fallible, and often harried, and it's up to you to protect your child from the consequences of the pressure they're under. Don't be intimidated by doctors or nurses. Demand information about the medications and treatments your child is getting, ask about the risks and side effects, be alert to sanitation deficiencies, and persist in asking your doctor to release your child as soon as possible.

Don't worry about being regarded as a nuisance by the hospital staff. That could be a useful reaction, because it may make them eager to send your child home!

21

How to Select the Right Doctor for Your Child

Now that you're aware of the hazards your child faces if he receives unnecessary or inappropriate medical treatment, you may be wondering how you can find a conscientious pediatrician and thus minimize the risks. How can you identify one who will treat your child properly when he needs treatment and tell you so candidly when he doesn't?

That's not an easy task, not so much because some doctors may be unethical or incompetent, but because of the system within which they are educated and function. To summarize what I have said earlier, you must never forget these points:

1. Doctors do what they have been trained to do. Although most childhood ailments will be cured by the body's own natural defenses, pediatricians are not trained to allow nature to take its course. They are trained to intervene, and all intervention is accompanied by risks to your child.

2. Unlike conscientious mechanics, who "don't fix what ain't broke," most doctors find it difficult to justify their fee for an office call if they tell you that your child doesn't need medical attention. They respond to perceived parental expectations by giving the child medicine

that is not required or tests that are not indicated and thus expose him to the risks that accompany virtually all drugs and many diagnostic procedures.

3. Although I've given it little attention in this book, doctors do have financial needs, particularly at the beginning of their careers, greater than those of almost any other profession. Most of them embark on their medical career heavily burdened with debt arising from their enormous education expenses and the costs of outfitting an office and must carry heavy office overhead from the very start. They have a strong, and in some cases irresistible, incentive to increase their income by providing services that your child doesn't need.

4. Increasingly, that incentive is compounded by growing competition within the medical profession. Doctors are emerging from the medical schools in record numbers, and in the areas in which most of them prefer to practice the demand for physicians no longer equals the supply. Responsible medical authorities project a surplus of 7,500 pediatricians by 1990. In order to maintain their incomes in the face of a dwindling supply of patients, doctors are impelled to increase the number of services provided to each of the patients who remains. This incentive will increase steadily in the years ahead.

This brings me back to the question I am most frequently asked: "How can I, as a concerned parent, select a conscientious pediatrician who will provide effective care but not overtreat my child?"

That's a perplexing question to which there is no pat answer. The standard advice given those seeking doctors is to consult the local medical society. They will give you a list of conveniently located pediatricians, but it won't tell you whether they are worth their salt, because the AMA does not measure the performance of its members. You will do as well by letting your fingers walk through the Yellow Pages.

My suggestion is that you begin your search by asking several of your friends what pediatricians or group practices they have used. Pick the one with whom a majority of them have established a rapport. That won't assure you of getting a competent, caring pediatrician who is not given to medical overkill, but it may improve the odds.

Once you have selected a doctor, observe closely his behavior during the time he spends with your child, keeping in mind what you have learned from this book. Here are the things you should watch for to determine whether the pediatrician you have selected is the right one for you.

1. Did he examine your child thoroughly and take a complete history during your first office visit?

2. Does he elicit from you on this and succeeding visits your observations about the physical and emotional condition of your child? That is a vital part of the history that no competent pediatrician should overlook.

3. When he asks a question, does he *listen* to what you have to say? Many doctors don't.

4. Does he answer your questions willingly, thoughtfully, and thoroughly, or does he brush them off and put you down?

5. Does he relate warmly to your child and win his confidence and affection almost at once?

6. Does he always hand you a prescription, or is he honest enough to admit it when he knows that nothing needs to be done for your child?

7. Does he explain thoroughly the hazards and side effects of the medications and immunizations that he prescribes?

8. Are your visits treated as perfunctory pill-peddling exercises, or does he display a genuine interest and counsel you on how to maintain the health of your child?

9. When you ask a question does he ever have the integrity to say, "I don't know?"

10. Does he respond promptly when an emergency requires that you call him on the phone?

Consider yourself lucky if you find the right doctor on your very first try. If the first pediatrician you visit falls short in any of the above respects, share your concern with him. If you've found the right doctor, he'll respect your candor and try to respond to your needs. If you haven't, find another doctor and try again. Before you have located the right one you may become as frustrated as Diogenes, but your child deserves any level of effort that is necessary to secure the most competent medical help that you can secure.

Don't fail to bear in mind, though, that it is you, not your doctor, who is the principal actor in preserving the health of your child. The right doctor will be able to help him when he is seriously ill, but you are the one with the opportunity and the responsibility to keep him well.

Author's References

Chapter 3

The shortcomings of "well-baby visits" are discussed in a commentary by Robert A. Hoekelman, M.D., Department of Pediatrics, University of Rochester, and references he cites, in *Pediatrics*, December 1980.

Chapter 4

For further information on the hazards of malnutrition in pregnancy see *What Every Pregnant Woman should Know: The Truth About Diets and Pregnancy*, by Gail S. Brewer and Tom Brewer, M.D., Random House, 1977.

Dr. Lewis Mehl's study of the "Statistical Outcomes of Home Birth in the United States" will be found in *Safe Alternatives in Childbirth*, by David Stewart, Ph.D., NAPSAC, Marble Hill, MO, 1976.

Concerns about the safety and value of diagnostic ultrasound are raised in Environmental Health Criteria Report No. 22, *Ultrasound*, published by the World Health Organization, Geneva, 1982. Also see the article, "Safe Form of Radiation Arouses New Worry," by Philip M. Boffey, *The New York Times*, August 2, 1983.

Chemical conjunctivitis in infants treated with silver nitrate is discussed in the *Merck Manual*, 14th edition, published by Merck, Sharp & Dohme.

The hazards and side effects of infant exposure to bilirubin lights were reported in 1979 by James Sidbury,

M.D., scientific director of the National Institute of Child Health and Human Development, Bethesda, MD. They are also discussed in the *Yearbook of Pediatrics*, 1977 and 1978, edited by Sydney S. Gellis, M.D.

The folly of exposing newborn babies to the risks of hexachlorophene baths was revealed in an assessment by N. M. Kanof, M.D., chairman of the American Medical Association Committee on Cutaneous Health and Cosmetics, in the *Journal of the American Medical Association (JAMA)*, 1972, Vol. 220, page 409: "There appears to be no need to apply any antibacterial agent to the cutaneous surface of the normal newborn infant. Contamination of nurseries can be controlled by the use of antibacterial agents on delivery room and equipment and personnel—the sources of infection." *Another reason to have your baby at home!*

The value of routine administration of vitamin K to newborn infants was discounted by Drs. J. M. Van Doorm, A. D. Muller, and H. C. Hemker in *The Lancet*, April 17, 1977: "We conclude that healthy babies, contrary to current beliefs, are not likely to have vitamin K deficiency . . . the administration of vitamin K to the newborn is not supported by our findings . . ."

The negative impact on breastfeeding of supplementary feeding of formula in the hospital nursery is described by Waldo Nelson, M.D., in the *Textbook of Pediatrics*, 7th Edition, Page 117: "Too much emphasis is put on daily weight gains. If early supplemental milk feedings are given to achieve this false goal, attempts at successful breastfeeding are doomed to failure, since it is usually easier for the infant to get milk from a bottle than from a breast."

Many studies indicate that maternal skin contact immediately after birth is as effective or more effective than placing the newborn in a radiant warmer. They include one by Hill and Shronk, *Journal of Obstetrics*, Sept./Oct. 1979, and another by J. Fardig, "A Comparison of Skin to Skin Contact and Radiant Heaters in Promoting Neonatal Thermoregulation," *Journal of Nurse/Midwifery*, Jan./Feb. 1980.

Chapter 5

Authorities who have noted the relationship between infant obesity and bottle-feeding with infant formula include Dr. Donald Naismith, a nutritionist at Queen Elizabeth Hospital, London; Dr. David M. Paige, of the Johns Hopkins School of Medicine, and many others. The relationship between infant and childhood obesity and adult obesity has also been extensively documented and was discussed fully by Dr. Simeon Margolies at an "obesity update" presented by the Johns Hopkins faculty.

Data on optimal weight gain during pregnancy, and its role in maternal milk production, was discussed in the *New England Journal of Medicine*, by Dr. George V. Mann, of Vanderbilt University, in 1974.

The incidence of malnutrition in hospitals has been widely reported in medical journals. Studies cited here were reported by Dr. Mark Raifman, director of pediatrics at Peninsula Hospital Center, Far Rockaway, N.Y., and Mary Price-Moissand, assistant professor in medical dietetics at the University of Illinois, at the annual meeting of the American Public Health Association.

Chapter 7

For further information on febrile convulsions see an article by Barton D. Schmitt, M.D., *American Journal of Diseases of Children*, February 1980, and "Prognosis in Children with Febrile Seizures," by Karin B. Nelson and Jonas H. Ellenberg, *Pediatrics*, May, 1978.

For a discussion of the consequences of long-term drug therapy to avoid febrile seizures see "Maintenance of Drug Therapy," by Dr. Samuel Livingston, et al, *Pediatric Annals*, April, 1979.

Chapter 10

"Antibiotic Use at Duke University Medical Center," a report on indiscriminate use of antibiotics in a hospital, by Mary Castle, RN, MPH, Catherine M. Wilfet, M.D., Thomas R. Cate, M.D., and Suydan Osterhout, M.D., was published in *JAMA*, June 27, 1977. It is but one of many similar studies at various hospitals throughout the country.

Further information on the "Misuse of Antibiotics for Treatment of Upper Respiratory Infections in Children" is contained in a report of the Clinical Pharmacology Unit, University of Vermont College of Medicine, published in *Pediatrics for the Clinician*, 1975. The incidence of side effects is also reported.

Chapter 11

The presence of streptococcal bacteria in the throats of 20 percent of school children is documented on page 246 of the 1982 report of the Committee on Infectious Diseases of the American Academy of Pediatrics.

Chapter 12

A critical study of the use of antibiotics and tympanostomy for treatment of ear infections was published in *The Lancet*, October 24, 1981. It reports on a double-blind study conducted by three Dutch physicians, F. L. Van Buchem, J. H. M. Dunk, and M. A. Van't Hof.

A study of the hazards of indiscriminate use of tympanostomy tubes for treatment of ear infection was reported in the *British Medical Journal* in 1981.

Chapter 13

The data on inappropriate prescribing of glasses for children and other deficiencies in pediatric care will be found in *Assessment of Medical Care for Children: Contrasts in Health Status, Vol. 3*, by David M. Kessner,

Carolyn Kalk Snow, and James Singer, Institute of Medicine, National Academy of Sciences, 1974.

Chapter 14

The disappointing results from dermabrasion treatment of acne scarring were reported by M. Spira, Baylor University College of Medicine, in *Plastic and Reconstruction Surgery*, July, 1977.

The statistical incidence of side effects from Accutane was reported in the *FDA Drug Bulletin*, July, 1983.

Chapter 15

The data on needless expenditures for shoes and the assertion that inexpensive canvas sneakers are adequate as basic shoes is from a report by Dr. Jeffrey Weiss, of Jefferson Medical College, Philadelphia, to the Ambulatory Pediatrics Association.

Chapter 16

Ray E. Helfer and Thomas L. Slovis of Michigan State University reported in 1977 a study of injuries suffered by children five or under who fell out of bed. In 80 percent of the cases there was no injury; 17 percent had minor bruises and scratches; only 3 percent sustained broken bones or fractured skulls that warranted medical attention, and there were no injuries that were life-threatening or permanently damaging to the child.

The high incidence of bone fractures among patients receiving steroid treatment for asthma was reported in a study conducted by Allen D. Adinoff, M.D., and J. Roger Hollister, M.D., of the National Asthma Center, Denver, CO.

Chapter 18

The 30-year study of the effect of psychological counseling on youths in Cambridge and Somerville, Mass., was reported at a meeting of the American Association of Psychiatric Services for Children in 1979. It was conducted by Joan McCord of Drexel University.

For further information on nutritional approaches to the treatment of mongolism see *Medical Treatment of Mongolism*, by Henry Turkel, M.D., in the Proceedings of the Second International Congress on Mental Retardation (Vienna, 1961), and *Can nutritional supplements help mentally retarded children: An exploratory study, Proceedings of the National Academy of Sciences*, USA, Vol. 70, January, 1981.

Chapter 19

Further documentation of the decline in incidence of several diseases prior to the introduction of vaccines can be found in "The Case Against Immunizations," by Richard Moskowitz, M.D., in the *Journal* of the American Institute of Homeopathy, March, 1983. Several significant studies are referenced.

The effects of vaccines on the immune response and other immunization issues are discussed in *Vaccinations and Immune Malfunctions*, by Harold E. Buttram, M.D., and John Chriss Hoffman, Humanitarian Publishing Company, Quakertown, PA, 1982.

The Los Angeles study of the relationship between DPT immunization and Sudden Infant Death Syndrome was conducted by Larry Baraff, M.D., et al, and is reported in *Pediatric Infectious Disease*, January, 1983.

A critique of the pertussis vaccine is contained in "Vaccination Against Whooping Cough: Efficiency vs. Risks," by Gordon T. Stewart, M.D., *The Lancet*, January, 1977. Further discussion of the risks and benefits of the DPT vaccine will be found in the paper, *Current Problems in Pediatrics*, issued by Vincent A. Fulginiti, M.D., University of Arizona College of Medicine, April, 1976.

A review of the value of breastfeeding in disease prevention is presented in the article, "Breastfeeding and the Prevention of Sudden Infant Death Syndrome," by

David A. Birnbaum, M.D., in the *Medical Trial Technique Quarterly*, Spring, 1978.

Details on the reluctance of California medical personnel to be vaccinated against rubella are reported in *JAMA*, February 20, 1981.

A report by Dr. Gordon T. Stewart on the Tennessee SIDS deaths following DPT immunization was published in *The Lancet*, August 18, 1979.

Chapter 20

Revealing studies of infections acquired in hospitals are discussed in *JAMA*, November 24, 1978, and in the article, "Hospital-Acquired Viral Respiratory Illness in a Pediatric Ward," *Pediatrics*, September, 1977.

The careless hand-washing habits of hospital personnel are the subject of a study, "Hand-Washing Patterns in Medical Intensive Care Units," *The New England Journal of Medicine*, June 11, 1981.

General References

Those interested in further information about the shortcomings of "medical science" are referred to these recent books:

Betrayers of the Truth: Fraud and Deceit in the Halls of Science, by William Broad and Nicholas Wade, Simon and Schuster, New York, 1982.

Health Shock: How to Avoid Ineffective and Hazardous Medical Treatment, by Martin Weitz, Prentice-Hall, New York, 1982.

Medicine Out of Control: The Anatomy of a Malignant Technology, by Richard Taylor, Sun Books, Melbourne, 1979.

INDEX

About the Author

ROBERT S. MENDELSOHN, M.D., has practiced pediatrics for over thirty years. A leading critic of modern medicine, he has helped stimulate significant improvements in the way medicine is practiced in the U.S. Dr. Mendelsohn's previous books include CONFESSIONS OF A MEDICAL HERETIC and MALE PRACTICE: HOW DOCTORS MANIPULATE WOMEN. This is his first book addressed to his own medical specialty.